EUROPEAN KINSHIP IN THE
AGE OF BIOTECHNOLOGY

Fertility, Reproduction and Sexuality

GENERAL EDITORS:

David Parkin, Director of the Institute of Social and Cultural Anthropology, University of Oxford

Soraya Tremayne, Co-ordinating Director of the Fertility and Reproduction Studies Group and Research Associate at the Institute of Social and Cultural Anthropology, University of Oxford, and a Vice-President of the Royal Anthropological Institute

Volume 1
Managing Reproductive Life: Cross-Cultural Themes in Fertility and Sexuality
Edited by Soraya Tremayne

Volume 2
Modern Babylon? Prostituting Children in Thailand
Heather Montgomery

Volume 3
Reproductive Agency, Medicine and the State: Cultural Transformations in Childbearing
Edited by Maya Unnithan-Kumar

Volume 4
A New Look at Thai AIDS: Perspectives from the Margin
Graham Fordham

Volume 5
Breast Feeding and Sexuality: Behaviour, Beliefs and Taboos among the Gogo Mothers in Tanzania
Mara Mabilia

Volume 6
Ageing without Children: European and Asian Perspectives on Elderly Access to Support Networks
Philip Kreager and Elisabeth Schröder-Butterfill

Volume 7
Nameless Relations: Anonymity, Melanesia and Reproductive Gift Exchange between British Ova Donors and Recipients
Monica Konrad

Volume 8
Population, Reproduction and Fertility in Melanesia
Edited by Stanley J. Ulijaszek

Volume 9
Conceiving Kinship: Assisted Conception, Procreation and Family in Southern Europe
Monica Bonaccorso

Volume 10
Where There is No Midwife: Birth and Loss in Rural India
Sarah Pinto

Volume 11
Reproductive Disruptions: Gender, Technology and Biopolitics In the New Millennium
Edited Marcia C. Inhorn

Volume 12
Reconceiving the Second Sex: Men, Masculinity, and Reproduction
Edited by Marcia C. Inhorn, Tine Tjørnhøj-Thomsen, Helene Goldberg and Maruska la Cour Mosegaard

Volume 13
Transgressive Sex: Subversion and Control in Erotic Encounters
Edited by Hastings Donnan and Fiona Magowan

Volume 14
European Kinship in the Age of Biotechnology
Edited by Jeanette Edwards and Carles Salazar

Volume 15
Kinship and Beyond: the Genealogical Model Reconsidered
Edited by Sandra Bamford and James Leach

Volume 16
Islam and New Kinship: Reproductive Technology and the Shariah in Lebanon
Morgan Clarke

EUROPEAN KINSHIP IN THE AGE OF BIOTECHNOLOGY

Edited by
Jeanette Edwards and Carles Salazar

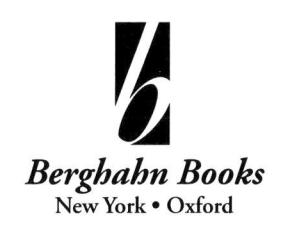

Berghahn Books
New York • Oxford

First published in 2009 by
Berghahn Books
www.berghahnbooks.com

©2009, 2012 Jeanette Edwards and Carles Salazar
First paperback edition published in 2012

All rights reserved. Except for the quotation of short passages for the purposes of criticism and review, no part of this book may be reproduced in any form or by any means, electronic or mechanical, including photocopying, recording, or any information storage and retrieval system now known or to be invented, without written permission of the publisher.

Library of Congress Cataloging-in-Publication Data

European kinship in the age of biotechnology / edited by Jeanette Edwards and Carles Salazar.
    p. cm. -- (Fertility, reproduction and sexuality ; v. 14)
Includes bibliographical references and index.
ISBN 978-1-84545-573-6 (hbk.) -- ISBN 978-0-85745-365-5 (pbk.)
  1. Kinship--Europe. 2. Artificial insemination, Human--Social aspects--Europe. 3. Human reproduction--Social aspects--Europe. I. Edwards, Jeanette, 1954- II. Salazar, Carles.

GN575.E93 2008
306.83094--dc22
                         2008052512

British Library Cataloguing in Publication Data

A catalogue record for this book is available from the British Library
Printed in the United States on acid-free paper.

ISBN: 978-0-85745-365-5 (paperback)

ISBN: 978-0-85745-650-2 (ebook)

Contents

Acknowledgements — vii

Introduction: The Matter in Kinship — 1
Jeanette Edwards

1. Knowing and Relating: Kinship, Assisted Reproductive Technologies and the New Genetics — 19
Joan Bestard

2. Imagining Assisted Reproductive Technologies: Family, Kinship and 'Local Thinking' in Lithuania — 29
Auksuolė Čepaitienė

3. Eating Genes and Raising People: Kinship Thinking and Genetically Modified Food in the North of England — 45
Cathrine Degnen

4. The Family Body: Persons, Bodies and Resemblance — 64
Diana Marre and Joan Bestard

5. The Contribution of Homoparental Families to the Current Debate on Kinship — 79
Anne Cadoret

6. Corpo-real Identities: Perspectives from a Gypsy Community — 97
Nathalie Manrique

7. Incest, Embodiment, Genes and Kinship — 112
Enric Porqueres i Gené and Jérôme Wilgaux

8. 'Loving Mothers' at Work: Raising Others' Children and Building Families with the Intention to Love and Take Care — 128
Enikő Demény

9. Adoption and Assisted Conception: One Universe of Unnatural Procreation. An Examination of Norwegian Legislation — 144
Marit Melhuus and Signe Howell

10. Fields of Post-human Kinship — 162
Ben Campbell

| **11.** | Are Genes Good to Think With?
Carles Salazar | 179 |

Notes on Contributors	197
Bibliography	201
Author Index	217
Subject Index	221

Acknowledgements

We gratefully acknowledge the support of the European Commission and would like to thank our desk officer, Alessio Vassarotti, for his efforts on our behalf. The editors would also like to thank Núria Montserrat Farré i Barril for her assistance in collating the bibliography, two anonymous referees for their careful reading of the manuscript and helpful suggestions, and Marie Rostron for administrive support and more. As coordinator of the project from which this volume stems, Jeanette Edwards would sincerely like to thank all members of the PUG team (the authors in this volume as well as Stéphane Bauzon, Catriona Bright, Cinzia Caporale, Darius Dauksas, Shahnaz Ibrahim, Gemma Orobitg, Júlia Ribot, Judit Sándor, Pat Spallone, Ildikó Takács, Katharine Tyler, Kari-Anne Ulfsnes and Peter Wade), who together created an intellectually stimulating, challenging and productive research environment the legacy of which is diffuse and enduring. She would also like to thank colleagues who participated in PUG workshops and in the final symposium, who engaged with our research with enthusiasm and generosity and from whom we learnt a great deal.

INTRODUCTION

The Matter in Kinship

Jeanette Edwards

'Public Understanding of Genetics': or PUG for Short

The chapters in this volume report on research carried out under the rubric of a project funded by the European Commission between 2002 and 2005. The project entailed a collaboration between scholars in France, Hungary, Lithuania, Italy, Norway, Spain and Britain and was conceived partly through a desire to investigate kinship, anthropologically, across Europe. It was clear from the ethnographic record that, while forms and practices of kinship differed markedly in different European contexts (see, for example, Strathern 1981; Gullestad 1984; Cohen 1987; Bestard 1991), there were interesting and unexplored resonances in how kin relatedness was conceptualised and in how persons were known to be 'made' and 'made up': to what extent was an empirical question. The research on which we report here aimed to look at kinship across Europe through the prism of the 'new genetics'. Partly this meant looking at the responses of various European 'publics' to new reproductive and genetic technologies (NRGT), but also, as the title of this volume suggests, it meant looking at kinship more broadly at a time when biotechnology specifically and molecular biology generally were prominent in the cultural imagination. Kinship was one theoretical thread, together with race and governance, of a larger project woven around the 'Public Understanding of Genetics' or PUG, for short (see also Wade 2007).[1]

PUG entailed a sustained conversation between anthropologists, historians, legal scholars and bioethicists.[2] For the anthropologists and anthropologically minded historians on the project, who have embraced, critiqued or at least been familiar with David Schneider's dictum, '[I]f science discovers new facts about biogenetic relationship, then that is what kinship is and was all along, although it may not have been known at the time' (1984: 23), it seemed self-evidently interesting to look at the relationship between kinship and new and burgeoning developments in genetic science and technology.[3] Interestingly kinship proved to be the most contested, albeit productively so, of the three theoretical strands in the project: partly because expertise in kinship was distributed amongst anthropologists (marked by distinctive and different European anthropological and ethnographic approaches to kinship) and non-anthropologists on the team. Indeed all 'publics' have an expertise in kinship and a major focus of this book is on the kinship expertise of a wide range of actors across several European countries. The publics who were the interlocutors in our research lived in rural and urban areas; in villages, towns and cities; they were patients, campaigners, legislators, clinicians, journalists, farmers, gardeners and others who, like many of the aforementioned, considered themselves to be 'just ordinary people'. They reflected, amongst other things, on significant and intimate social relationships; on what is required to grow 'proper' persons; on how family ties are created, maintained and broken; on the difference between family and kin; on the politics of knowledge; and on the interrelatedness of human and non-human lives. The nature of the kind of kinship thinking they mobilised allows for, or even encourages, contestation. It entails the interplay of a myriad of factors, some of which are given and others acquired, some fixed and others mutable, some located in the domain of nature and others in society and with certain factors (and not others) foregrounded at any given moment. In the concluding chapter of this volume, Carles Salazar unpacks further the analytical approaches to these rich and diverse ethnographic data. Here I note the sticking points: the points from which we (as analysts) found it difficult to dislodge ourselves.

Of Newness and Novelty

There have been a number of recent and well-cited publications in English that have excavated particular histories of anthropological kinship theory. They all remark on the rising, declining and re-emerging significance of kinship in social and cultural anthropology during the twentieth century and point to a rupture between 'the old' kinship studies and 'the new' (see, for example, Holy 1996; Carsten 2000a, 2004; Faubion 2001; Franklin and McKinnon 2001; Parkin and Stone 2004).[4] They identify a rekindling of anthropological interest in kinship which has been partly fuelled by the challenge and opportunity posed by emerging 'alternative' or 'new' family forms in many Western societies, some of which, but by no means all, have been facilitated by developments in biotechnology.[5] Anthropologists have increasingly turned their attention to 'Euro-American' kinship with studies on, amongst other things, reconstituted, adopted and stepfamilies (for example, Stacey 1991; Modell 1994; Simpson 1994, 1998; Howell 2003), lesbian and gay kinship (for example, Weston 1991; Lewin 1993; Hayden 1995; Cadoret 2003) and new reproductive technologies (NRT), including gamete donation and surrogate motherhood (for example, Ragoné 1994; Franklin 1997; Thompson 2001; Melhuus 2003; Konrad 2005). The novelty of particular reproductive technologies is a moot point and the epithet 'new' is clearly not only, or predominantly, a marker in time, nor does it merely reflect the novelty of particular practices or technologies, although it might embrace both these things.[6] It is as much a perspective, an angle from which the contemporary world is perceived, and defining something as 'new' both opens up a vista and occludes what came before.

Novelty is an endemic aspect of a current Zeitgeist in which science and technology are understood to be creating radical social change and decisive breaks with the past; within a world at once smaller (globalised) and speeded up. The ascendancy of biological and information technologies and their intervention in 'life itself' are said to have removed what were thought to be the stable underpinnings of a given nature. Marilyn Strathern dates the shift to the end of the modern epoch, when nature no longer provided 'the model or analogy for the very idea of context' (1992a: 195) on which and from which the plurality of individuals and their societies could be imagined. As the possibilities of, and reflection upon, human intervention in nature increased and nature could increasingly be seen to be both manipulated and manipulable, then, it lost its grounding function. For some, Strathern over-states her case. Peter Wade (2002) remarks that the plastic and performative aspects of human nature in Western thought predates the modernist epoch, while Enric Porqueres i Gené and Jérôme Wilgaux (this volume) take issue with what they see as the incommensurability between Western and non-Western concepts of nature implied in Strathern's argument. However, each acknowledges, in different ways, that the character and 'make-up' of nature has, nevertheless, changed. The point remains that, as developments in biotechnology applied to human procreation continue apace, the explicitness they provoke about the component parts of both kinship and personhood brings to mind aspects of each that remained implicit when boxed into the realm of nature.

The 'new kinship studies' have been driven by at least two major imperatives. The first can be seen in the concerted attempt by anthropologists to put social aspects of kinship on the map. A reaction against the privileging of biology and what was perceived as the fixity of the genealogical grid, the aim was, in part, to critique and question any remaining and lurking biological determinism in kinship definitions. Anthropologists were keen to show through ethnographic example how social connection was as significant as (and in some cases more significant than) biological connection. Through this process the notion of 'fictive kinship' was rejected and shown to be an ideological construction that did little justice to ethnographic realities. As in earlier studies of kinship, 'the biological' was bracketed off and deemed outside or beyond the concern of anthropology of a social or cultural bent. While it might be given, and even thought axiomatically to be part of kinship, biology was deemed not nearly as interesting, or political, or revealing, as ways in which social ties are forged and sustained through, for example, feeding, caring and proximity. The latter were considered the 'proper' focus of anthropological attention even if in European conceptions social ties were still forged through what are considered to be biological ideologies such as those of 'shared blood' (a point to which I return).

The second impetus came from a burgeoning ethnographic interest in science and its technologies. Anthropologists turned their attention to those elements of kinship deemed biological and 'un-bracketed' them. Drawing on studies that looked ethnographically and historically at the anatomical and physiological bodies and body parts of biomedicine (e.g. Laqueur 1990; Martin 1991, 1994; Oudshoorn 1994), they remarked on the way in which gametes and hormones, for example, have social and gendered properties and how bio-scientific discourse draws on wider cultural understandings in constituting the materials and objects of its study. Western scientific models and categories and the idioms used to explain human reproduction, for example, became a legitimate focus of anthropological enquiry, and anthropologists drew fruitfully on and engaged with the burgeoning field of science and technology studies (STS) in a focus on the culturally constructed body. In anthropological theorising about 'Western' kinship, the limits to constructivist accounts became apparent as what got to be included as biological remained notably under-problematised.[7]

What both these impetuses (artificially separated out in this commentary) have in common is a tendency to keep the domains of 'the biological' and 'the social' (also artificially separated out in commentary) intact and separate.[8] Ethnographically, however, it is not always predictable what aspects of kinship will get slotted into each and indeed the distinction between the two is not always clear-cut. As one is made more explicit, so too is the other: to what extent can they be unhitched? We need to ask in all seriousness whether our informants are placing certain elements of kinship in a 'biology box' and others in a 'social box' or whether we, as analysts, are doing it for them. How far, in other words, do we too readily locate certain elements of kinship in what we deem to be the realm of biology? This is an old, thorny and perennial anthropological question, and without wishing to return to arguments about the relationship between emic and etic categories (well rehearsed by Gellner 1973 and Needham 1971, for example; with excellent overviews by Harris 1990 and Holy 1996; and see Strathern 2005), it behoves us to acknowledge the tension. Our interest here is in the way in which 'the biological' and 'the social' themselves get (re)produced through the conceptualisation and enactment of kinship.

Just as problematic as the idea that 'everything is new', with attendant images of a radical rupture between the past and the present, is the idea that nothing is. There can be no doubt that developing and burgeoning technologies of communication, science, medicine, bureaucracy, surveillance, information, enhancement and so on have created particular conditions of possibility. The question is whether the contemporary 'newness', recognised acutely in formative and intimate relations of kinship, reflects changes in epistemology as well as practice. 'New family forms' and 'new studies of kinship' are deeply implicated in each other but how indicative they are of what Janet Carsten (2004) identifies as 'new forms of kinship' is an ethnographic question. The studies from which this volume draws show 'old' idioms of kinship to be remarkably resilient, albeit put to work in unpredictable and unexpected ways. They also show 'new' idioms of kinship being put to work in ways that are decidedly familiar.

The chapter by Porqueres i Gené and Wilgaux in this volume exemplifies the tenacity of prior meanings and the plasticity of familiar idioms. In a historical analysis of incest prohibitions in Europe, Porqueres i Gené and Wilgaux compare the use of 'blood' and 'genes' in explanations for why sexual intercourse between specific categories of kin is prohibited. They show that, while genetic explanation is increasingly given as a reason for avoiding incest, there are noticeable and notable similarities between contemporary 'genes' and ancient 'blood': both act as 'programmers' and blood, they argue, was not so different from genes in its ability to transmit and communicate particular characteristics. The authors show the importance of a historical approach to kinship and they caution against arguments that posit a radical shift in European kinship. I am struck in this chapter by the way in which the contemporary, in this case 'the gene', provides an analytical handle on the past and on the familiar and enduring idiom of 'blood'. The analysis works both ways.

The chapters in this volume address questions about what is new in both kinship as it is 'done' and kinship as it is analysed. They draw on studies from both 'old' and 'new' Europe and are influenced by 'old' and 'new' kinship theory: they interrogate the trend to newness itself.[9] The authors report on research with lesbian families in France, with foster-mothers in Hungary, with families created through transnational adoption in Norway and Spain, through new reproductive technologies in Catalonia, and through feeding in England; they draw on fieldwork in rural and urban communities in Spain, Lithuania and England; and on research in organisations and in clinics, with archival material and documents and on the Internet. They necessarily engage critically with 'old' and 'new' anthropological theorising in order to do justice to the creativity with which kinship is 'done' in their fieldwork sites. They embrace conventions of 'new' ethnography with studies that are translocal and multi-sited, while locating their work in both 'old' and 'new' disciplinary trajectories building and reflecting on a variety of analytical and anthropological traditions. Trained in, amongst other things, ethnology under Soviet (pre)occupations, structuralism in the manner of Levi-Strauss or genealogical methods from W.H.R. Rivers, their studies are also inflected by feminist and postmodern critique. Many carried out their first fieldwork in cultures considered to be 'traditional' domains of social anthropology, others continued national traditions of anthropology 'at home', while others bucked the trend, whatever it was.

In Europe

As Anne Cadoret remarks in this volume, it still appears to be difficult to write about anthropological kinship without reference to Schneider. He is often located at the fault line between the past and the present and credited, or blamed, depending on which way you look at it, with a so-called revolution in the anthropological study of kinship.[10] According to Linda Stone, he 'dropped a bomb on the field of anthropology' (Parkin and Stone 2004: 241); and 'the bomb', according to her, was his revelation that kinship, as anthropologists had previously understood it, was a European folk model based on biological connection and sexual reproduction.[11]

There are at least two conceptual legacies from Schneider that continue to trouble. The first is 'Euro-American' and the second 'biogenetic'. I shall return to the second below. For Schneider, 'Euro-American' is partly a way of distinguishing white North Americans of European ancestry from 'Afro-Americans', 'Asian Americans', 'Native Americans' and so on. In his early work on American kinship and in the distinction he posits between cultural and normative levels, he juxtaposes Western, European and North American cultural systems. His informants were white, middle-class Americans from a range of European backgrounds and predominantly Protestant, Catholic or Jewish (and see Stone 2000). While later he was to acknowledge the impact of ethnicity and class on American kinship, the idea of Euro-American as a cultural system proved resilient, even if it had to be constantly problematised and the epithet Anglo added. If one effect of the idiom was to differentiate, it was also used to aggregate: to reflect what are thought to be resonances between European and North American world views. It has also been taken up to mark similarity between particular European and North American ideologies (and cosmologies (Strathern 2005) and again as a proxy for Western. It has been used usefully to refer to a discourse of science, governance and bureaucracy not confined to North America or Europe, or 'uniform within them' (Strathern 2005: 163), but nevertheless, many would argue, increasingly hegemonic.

One aim of much recent anthropological work on kinship has been to reformulate it in ways that 'escape' a Euro-American cultural bias. But, all too often, implicit in this formulation are assumptions about precisely what Euro-American kinship looks like.[12] The privileging of biology (and connected to this the ubiquity of 'blood' and the emerging dominance of 'the gene') is often considered to be a key defining feature of it. Undoubtedly, in specific contexts the transmission and sharing of biogenetic substance are emphasised as the source of kinship, but this is not the only way in which kinship is conceptualised. An understanding of kinship as ultimately based in biology is neither sufficient nor complex enough to deal with the ethnographic reality across Europe, let alone across Europe and North America. For Cadoret (this volume), and the lesbian parents in France about whom she writes, naming strategies, for example, establish and affirm the relationship between each parent (two mothers) and their child (and see also the chapter by Melhuus and Howell). This does not necessarily entail cutting out as insignificant the tie between their child and its genitor who is not 'called upon' to be a parent on a daily basis, but of putting the connection in its place as one among others. The concept of plural kinship developed by Cadoret includes biology as one particular 'truth', but no more or less 'truthful' than those other activities required to 'reproduce' a human person, such as 'feeding the child, rearing it, providing a name [and] transmitting status'.

Cathrine Degnen's chapter picks up and expands on the theme of feeding. The English mothers with whom she spoke feel keenly their parental responsibility to monitor the food their children eat. The kind of food their children ingest reflects not only their responsibility as a parent but also their capacity for creating particular kinds of children. By bringing together technologies not usually brought together, Degnen fruitfully shows what an analysis of people's responses to genetically modified food (GMF) can add to insights that have been gained through the analysis of technologies applied to human reproduction.

'Euro-American' is the kind of shorthand that proves valuable when trying to discern a world view that deploys and promotes a language of science and bureaucracy appropriated across national and geographical boundaries, but is a hindrance when attached to particular populations and real lives. Together, the chapters in this volume manage to maintain the tension between the generalisable and the idiosyncratic. Familiar themes and motifs run through the different studies and there is evidence of sensibilities and imaginaries not confined within country borders: across a range of publics, similar symbolic threads are woven in familiar ways.[13] At the same time, however, there is evidence of intriguing differences. If we consider, for example, legislation and policy as a site of kinship (as a site in which certain kinship understandings are crystallised, albeit perhaps temporarily and often controversially), then the differences between the countries in which we have been working are revealing. If we take the substitution of gametes in fertility treatment as one simple example, then we see a notable lack of standardisation in legislative and policy responses. In Norway legislation does not permit the donation of ova, in Britain it is allowed under licence, while in Spain it is allowed, as is explicit advertising to recruit egg donors.[14]

If novel ways of forming families in Western contexts have inspired fresh approaches to kinship, questions about the extent to which anthropological kinship theory is coterminous with a particular 'folk model' (which, as we know, for Schneider (1968) was European and for Bouquet (1993) British) remain. Drawing on ethnographic examples from across Europe, the authors in this collection interrogate the European 'folk model' that was meant to have informed anthropological kinship theory and which anthropologists were accused of exporting around the world and applying to kinship systems that did not rely on the same premises. They introduce examples of explicit discussion and formulation of kinship and of what matters. The title of this volume, *European Kinship*, points to the range of kinship undertakings it addresses and the title of this introduction to the fact that kinship *matters*, both ethnographically and analytically (and see Ebtehaj et al. 2006). It also nods to the materiality – 'the matter' – of kinship, which, as you will see, interests many of the contributors to this collection.

The chapters in this collection contribute to discussion about what might be gained and what might be lost when the focus is on both 'Euro-American' and the contemporary in the study of kinship. The majority of the informants in the ethnographic studies reported here are white Europeans. They belong to different social classes and claim diverse European origins and national identities.[15] They reveal similarities and differences across European sites, and importantly across time, in cosmologies that include kinship.

In Kinship

Although held directly responsible, by some, for the demise of kinship in anthropology from the 1970s to the 1990s and indirectly responsible for its revival in the early 1990s (Stone 2004), Schneider was developing arguments that were also being made elsewhere. Although he alleged that 'his predecessors and contemporaries were mired in a genealogical way of thinking that rested, if only tacitly, on a view of kinship as ultimately biological' (Parkin and Stone 2004: 19), the debate, mentioned above, foreshadowed Schneider's critique. The relationship between kinship as an analytical construct and kinship 'on the ground' – or kinship as a figment of the anthropological imagination and an empirical reality – had already been hotly debated (and see Harris 1990).[16] There are many commentaries on Schneider's critique, not least his own reflections (Schneider 1995; see also Feinberg and Ottenheimer 2001), and it may seem excessive to add yet more. But, as we noted earlier, a collection of chapters such as this which draws on ethnographic examples from across Europe has the potential of shedding some light on the question of which 'indigenous view' or 'European folk model' it is that is coterminous with the model Schneider accused anthropologists of exporting around the world.[17] The authors of this volume are neither mired in a genealogical way of thinking, nor do they glibly conflate genealogy and biology, but they are nevertheless interested ethnographically in when and where genealogical and biological understandings of kinship are conflated and where biological relatedness is and is not privileged.

The chapter by Marit Melhuus and Signe Howell brings the countervailing and contradictory tendencies in contemporary European kinship into focus. Again bringing into the same analysis social practices not usually brought together, in their case transnational adoption and assisted reproductive technologies, and by tracking historically the shifts that have occurred in legislation on both, they present evidence of an increasing 'biologisation' of kin relatedness in Norway – and this at the same time as evidence of broader public understandings of the way in which kin relatedness is forged through different kinds of social intimacies (what Howell (2006) describes as a process of 'kinning'). In their chapter on transnational adoption in Spain, Diana Marre and Joan Bestard present intriguing examples of how family resemblance is used to forge kinship ties without biological ties (as narrowly conceived). Their material provocatively questions narrow conceptions of biological relatedness by showing the way in which physical bonds are forged and baby bodies placed firmly into the body of the family through what is seen to be familiar.

If, as Strathern (1992a) notes, kinship is a hybrid connecting the domains of nature and culture, it belongs in neither one nor the other. But the danger is that the (re)focus on the social aspects of kinship firms up the distinction between the 'biological' and 'social' and focusing on the boundaries between the two leaves them intact (see Carsten 2000a). Is the interplay between 'the biological' and 'the social' of a piece with the interplay between nature and culture? How readily can biology be mapped on to the domain of nature? Can they effortlessly stand in for each other? In the European contexts on which we focus here, people constantly remark on what they consider to be natural and, in that sense, what belongs to the domain of nature; there are some practices and materials they consider more natural than others. Nature, as we know is neither stable nor fixed, and kinship is a key site in which distinctions between nature and culture, what is given and what is acquired, what is fixed and what is changeable, are produced. The European citizens whose ideas and understandings we report in this volume frequently mobilise nature in their rendering of kinship. They also naturalise – place into the domain of nature – non-biological elements of relatedness.

Let's look at 'blood'. Long analysed as an element of a biological ideology, can 'blood' be contained within the biological domain? It appears to spill over and, in marking kinship, its excesses connect it to a range of kin. An English woman, in her early sixties, echoes many of her compatriots when she tells me that a child born through surrogacy arrangements will still be part of the surrogate mother even if the surrogate has not provided the egg. In her words:

> It's got that surrogate mother's blood – the foetus feeds off the blood supply of the mother – off the person who is carrying the child – so that mother's blood is still going through that surrogate baby's veins. So it's never truly the parent's – it's always part of the donor's blood scheme, isn't it? They always say 'blood's thicker than water'. (cited in Edwards 2004: 770)

The idioms in which this woman explores the possibility and potential of gestational surrogacy are telling: the surrogate mother, in her example, is the 'donor', and the baby is a 'surrogate' who does not belong only and wholly to its parents. These idioms draw our attention to the surrogate relationship between the baby and its surrogate mother and the way in which her blood leaves a trace in the baby that can never be fully removed: it is enduring – because, as we all know, she suggests, 'blood is thicker than water'.

Listen to what one Lithuanian woman told Čepaitienė about the same kind of surrogacy arrangement:[18] 'the only input in that case, is the fact that the child develops in that woman's body. But it would still be affected by certain hormones, it would still bond [with her].' This woman remarks on the bond forged between a woman and the fetus she gestates, with or without a genetic connection. For her the substance that constitutes the tie between the surrogate mother and the child she gestates is hormonal: the bond is made explicit and substantiated in hormones. Commenting on this view, and others like it, Čepaitienė notes that the child is thought inevitably to contain a portion of the woman who carries and gives birth to it. In Lithuania, she continues, 'blood' is neither a fixed nor a predictable quality.

In a similar vein, Nathalie Manrique traces the resonances and affinities between Gypsy conceptualisations of kinship and what counts as evidence of relatedness and scientific and, more precisely, biogenetic understandings of relatedness – both, she argues, are wedded to verifiable facts. For the Gypsies of Morote and San Juan in Spain, 'blood' is gendered and comes in different strengths. Thus the offspring of a Gypsy woman and *Payo* (non-Gypsy) man is undoubtedly Gypsy, because '[t]he male, active property of the Gypsy woman's blood during her menstruation is ... stronger than the *Payo* blood'.

Perhaps it is useful to keep in mind this multivalency of 'blood' when we think about the place of genetics and genealogy in contemporary European kinship. While Melhuus and Howell remark that in Norway '"blood" has become limited to biogenetic relations and denotes "origin" and "identity", irrespective of the social relations involved', other studies show that genetic connection is not coterminous with genealogical connection, and 'blood' does not fully map on to genetics, just as it does not fully map on to biology: blood and biological connection are not necessarily coterminous (and see Manrique, this volume). Talk of blood and bloodlines cannot automatically be reduced to biological explanation, and indeed biological explanation is not axiomatically reductionist – blood is thick with condensed meaning even if it is not always, or everywhere, 'thicker than water'. The notion of shared blood as constituting relatedness is powerful, but it cannot axiomatically be reduced to either the biogenetic specifically or to biology more generally. It is symbolically and metaphorically powerful and as such we, as analysts, should resist the attempt to purify it – to draw out of it one congealed meaning – while at the same time showing ethnographically where and how this happens.

It has become a truism, not least through innovative and insightful social, historical and philosophical studies of science (e.g. Haraway 1991, 1997; Latour 1991; Knorr-Cetina 1999; Jasanoff 2004), that science does not merely reflect but also constitutes its subject of study.[19] And, in so far as it too is deeply embedded in, and reflective of, the societies that sponsor it as an academic endeavour, social anthropology is no different in that respect. At the same time, however, it has to contend seriously with the preoccupations of those it studies, who also theorise about the worlds in which they live. The contemporary explicitness with which kin relatedness and what constitutes it are rendered visible and made available to scrutiny reveals the premises and assumptions from which understandings of kinship are built, and consequently what is at stake when they are contested.

Metaphorical bombs are perhaps, then, too loud an image with which to portray the subtle shifts of emphasis emerging in recent anthropological studies of kinship. If the sheer volume of recently published anthropological works on kinship is anything to go by, then Schneider's call to abolish 'kinship' (Schneider 1984) has gone unheeded, and so too has the call to replace the discredited idiom with a broader concept of 'relatedness' (Carsten 2000a). Instead, facilitated by ethnographic scrutiny of Western, European or even 'Euro-American' models of kinship that anthropologists were accused of exporting around the world, the kinship concept has survived. The authors in this volume have not eschewed kinship, but instead have broadened and strengthened it and put it to work in ways that do justice to their ethnographic examples.

In Biotechnology

Many social commentators have identified the potentially reductive impulse in biotechnology. In idioms of geneticisation, biologisation and (bio)medicalisation, social scientists have attempted to capture its impact on cultural understandings of, for example, health and healing, the body and its disorders and kinship and inheritance (e.g. Lippman 1992; Finkler 2000, 2001).[20] Recent critiques of the 'geneticisation' thesis turn on complexity and contingency within the biological sciences, acknowledged by biologists and geneticists themselves (see Franklin 2001; and contributors to McKinnon and Silverman 2005, especially Taussig), and on the uneven and unpredictable impact of medical genetics on those directly affected.[21] Katie Featherstone and her colleagues in Cardiff, for example, write of the wider consequences for kin of an individual either diagnosed with or discovered to be 'at risk' of a specific genetic disorder and the complex and difficult negotiations they face over what to reveal and to whom (Featherstone et al. 2006). The dilemmas facing people undergoing genetic testing are clearly acute and test results inevitably bring to mind connections that are traced along genetic lines, which then may have to be acted upon. For Featherstone et al. the conflation of genetic technologies and reproductive technologies is ultimately unhelpful. They argue that, while reproductive technologies have weakened the link between the 'biological facts of conception and the social categories of kinship', the new genetics (referring to the development of genetic tests to diagnose and predict an increasing number of medical conditions) strengthens the 'conventional categories of reproduction and biological relatedness' (Featherstone et al. 2006: 6). The point is well taken. Nevertheless, it also shows precisely why it is helpful to bring disparate applications of biotechnology together. Doing so reveals a kinship thinking that is characterised by both fixed and manipulable aspects and where one or the other can be, and is, foregrounded.[22] Our own point of departure is that they inform each other and placing them alongside one another provokes analogies and connections that illuminate rather than obscure. As mentioned above, Melhuus and Howell in this volume juxtapose new reproductive technologies and transnational adoption as part of the same 'procreative universe'. They also find two opposing trends: 'one that privileges the biological over the social (NRT) and the other that privileges, albeit somewhat uneasily, the social over the biological (adoption)'. Degnen's chapter shows convincingly how an analysis of the way in which genetically modified foods (GMF) are understood, which in her cases focuses on the intersection of 'genes, body and food', can inform and be informed by what we know about the way in which genetic technologies for human therapeutic purposes are understood. The point to make is that the kind of kinship that emerges through the ethnographic window of NRT, transnational adoption, fostering or GMF is characterised by precisely the two elements that Featherstone and colleagues identify: a relatedness anchored in and to biology (and not only biology) and a relatedness unanchored (buoyant but not necessarily more ebullient). Contributors to this volume are interested in the way in which kinship across Europe embraces both immutability and plasticity: connection traced through genes, for example, is accompanied by connection traced through affection and either one of them might assume priority depending on the context, that is, depending on the reason that specific connections are being traced. It is not clear, however, that the biological is the fixed (and somehow more sedate) pole in this duality and the social the 'movable feast'.[23]

While it might now be a truism to say that kinship can no longer be understood as the cultural elaboration of 'natural facts', or that 'biology' can no longer be bracketed off as of no anthropological consequence, what we should include as 'natural fact' or what we should put into the biological bag is not self-evident. Sarah Franklin argues that the dramatic shifts occurring in the 'new biologies' belie any simple understanding of them as providing fixed, rigid or constraining models. In her words: 'Biotechnology is today the matrix of unprecedented life-forms that have as little to do with the nature of biology once depicted as they do with the biology portrayed by Schneider' (Franklin 2001: 320). For her, the 'new biologies' are the 'material-semiotic practices of the contemporary biological sciences', which together with the 'new biologicals ... new entities such as cryopreserved human embryos, cloned transgenic animals, genetically modified seeds and patented gene sequences' means that biology is constantly making itself 'strange' (Franklin 2001: 303, 320). If this is the case, we need to be more aware about the tendency to stereotype it as some kind of fixed and essentialising understanding of the natural world (see also Nash 2002). Having said that, the authors in this volume show, ethnographically, when and how the concept of biology is used to do precisely that: when it is used to signify a fixed and essential substratum to social life. The chapters in this collection show the kind of work the biology concept is made to do. While the authors here question any simple reduction of biology to genetics, they also show what in different contexts gets to be biological and how it is put to work.

What to Keep Steady

> You cannot have a public debate without holding *some* of the terms steady – whereas in the real world nothing stays still and it is likely that the terms with which we speak are not just evolving but *co*-evolving in relation to one another. (Strathern 2004: 53, original emphasis)

An argument about kinship means keeping certain terms steady. One approach, exemplified by Salazar (in this volume) is to keep 'the gene' and a scientific understanding of genetic inheritance steady: as universally instrumental in the production of life 'as we know it'. Then the task is to discern empirically where and when genetics is relevant (or not) in the creation and constitution of persons. Salazar invites us to hold a scientific explanation steady and to show through our different projects how 'genetic knowledge' is made socially relevant. The aim is to see how scientific knowledge (in this case of genetics) travels, how it is translated and transformed. Salazar maintains a theoretical tension between scientific (biogenetic) and social (kinship) knowledge, and furnishes us with a further set of generative dichotomies: syntagmatic and paradigmatic relations; scientific and lay knowledge (or cognitive systems); truth and symbolic knowledge and so on.[24] His analysis is explicitly structural.[25] And our task, from this perspective, is to excavate the system of cultural meanings that 'depend on each other for their validation, and not on the "real" objects they presumably refer to' (Salazar, this volume). He concludes that kinship thinking deposits meaning on genetics (and conversely genetics deposits meaning on kinship) and that genes (as kinship entities like 'blood', 'flesh' or 'bones') are relational not substantial. This echoes the findings of Porqueres i Gené and Wilgaux (this volume), who show that the transmission of 'blood' (prior to the use of genetic idioms) was never only about the transmission and sharing of substance.

Enikő Demény describes, with empathy, the role of professional foster-mothers in Hungary. A condition of their employment is that they live alone in the SOS Children's Villages where they work and, despite the valuable role they play in the lives of children in the care of the state, they have to negotiate and deal with dominant ideologies that not only validate biological motherhood but also denigrate the family unit without a male head. Demény reveals the tension between their roles as 'loving mothers' and as paid workers. While drawing on concepts from psychology and psychoanalytical theory to explain how foster-mothers 'internalise' the dominant discourse, her material also shows us how techniques of signification, communication and technologies of the self (Foucault 1981, cited in Borneman 1992) produce particular subjectivities. The explicitness with which kinship is explained, reflected upon, made and denied by the publics with whom we have worked in this research is noteworthy. However, the more a process of 'geneticisation' or 'biocentrism' occurs, the more noticeable is desire, or affective ties or invention. An intentionality and agency in the making, breaking and sustaining of intimate social relations emerges from the empirical projects reported here: an intentionality that recalls Strathern's comments on debates over NRT, where 'an increasing emphasis on corporalisation (biology)' is accompanied by 'an increasing value given to conceptual or mental effort. Thus what are constantly (re)created as the underlying realities of genetic makeup are counterbalanced by the accord given to human invention' (Strathern 1999: 21).

Another approach in a debate about kinship might be to keep relationality steady. The kinship thinking our projects reveal is noticeable in its oscillation (relationship) between 'the biological' and 'the social'. Our projects show where one is emphasised over and above the other to the extent that the other is not only undermined but screened out. There is a constant movement between the significance and insignificance, the foregrounding and backgrounding, the emphasis and underestimation of biological connection. It is partisan to take either the social or the biological as indicative and definitive of kinship.[26] But ethnographically that is what happens all the time. Europe expert bioethical debate, for example, hones in on the 'rights' of children conceived with donated sperm to 'know' their biological fathers, and social workers in Norway insist on the links between transnational adoptees and their biological kin. At the same time, lesbian couples in France make claims on French rules of cognatic kinship to firm up their parental connection with their children conceived with donated semen (Cadoret, this volume) and young mothers in the north of England insist that their stepfather is the grandfather of their children (Edwards 2005). In these examples, from amongst many we could cite, either 'nature' or 'nurture' or biological or social ties are privileged (foregrounded). But the point to reiterate is that they rely on each other for their purchase: it is the interplay between the two that is the significant characteristic of this kind of kinship.

Joan Bestard's chapter suggests an escape from the pendulum. Drawing on social actor network theory (ANT), he invites us to think of kinship as emerging from a network of heterogeneous entities, which might include 'gametes, donors, parents, names, localities, identities and properties'. For Bestard, thinking of kinship in terms of 'networks of unrelated entities' militates against deterministic models, be they biological or social, and better reflects his ethnographic data in fertility clinics in Spain, which reveal people creating and mobilising complex moral landscapes.

Identified by Cadoret (1995; and this volume) as 'plural', it is precisely the plurality of the kinship we are interested in here that gives it its creative and generative properties. It makes and connects a whole range of persons, to each other, to places and to pasts, and indeed, as Ben Campbell argues in this volume, it connects human and non-human worlds. Campbell's chapter shows beautifully the way in which the non-human world – the birds and 'wee beasties', as well as the flora and fauna of the English countryside – is enlisted in English kinship thinking. He uses British responses to genetically modified organisms (GMO), played out in the media, to decentre what he sees as the humancentric bias in the anthropology of kinship. For him, 'genetic knowledge of humans, non-humans and humanly modified organisms re-situates how we can think of ourselves relationally to the non-human world'.

Rather than an increasing uncertainty and unease about kinship (Carsten 2004) we find, ethnographically, a confidence and in some sense a lack of doubt about who is to be considered kin. There may be diverse ways in which French lesbian couples create a family – from where they procure semen, how they each relate and intend to relate to their child, who they choose as sperm donor and the role they intend for him in their family – but their relatedness to their children is not in doubt. Kin connections can be traced in a number of registers, for example, through substance, affection, spirit or legislation. A plural kinship system is one where different ways of imagining kin connection are available and readily mobilised. It is the plurality itself that is of theoretical interest. The question remains as to whether, as Ladislav Holy argues, kinship 'has to be understood as a culturally specific notion of relatedness deriving from shared bodily and/or spiritual substance and its transmission' (Holy 1996: 171; see also Héritier 1994; Porqueres i Gené and Wilgaux, this volume).[27]

This book brings together things that are rarely brought together. It brings together ethnographic studies from across Europe that focus on the way in which kinship is forged, imagined, sustained and denied. It places different kinds of biotechnology in the same frame and places them alongside practices that are far from biotechnological. It also brings together different approaches to the study of kinship, which appear to glance off of each other but which, on second glance, speak to each other in fruitful, and unexpected, ways.

Notes

1. Public Understanding of Genetics: a Cross-cultural and Ethnographic Study of the 'New Genetics' and Social Identity (PUG), Quality of Life and Management of Living Resources Programme, Framework 5: contract no. QLG 7–CT–2001–01668. http://www.socialsciences.manchester.ac.uk/pug/index.htm.
2. An enterprise that brought together academics working in seven different European countries and also at different stages in their career inevitably revealed the strikingly different institutional conditions in which academic

work is pursued within Europe, as well as distinctive conventions of collaboration and scholarship.
3. Schneider made the mutuality of the scientific and Western folk model of kinship explicit. If it is the case that kinship is whatever science discovers about biogenetic connection, we would expect developments in genetic technologies to impact on kinship thinking.
4. It could be argued that from French perspectives kinship never went out of fashion and a lineage from Claude Lévi-Strauss to Françoise Héritier bypasses Schneider 'continuing a long-standing French interest in filiation, alliance and incest' (Edwards 2008).
5. Alternative, that is, to models of the 'nuclear' family, where biological and social parenthood were supposed to be coterminous and which in itself was an ideal that was never the only way in which families were 'made up'.
6. Pregnancies have been achieved through donor insemination in the UK since the 1950s (and see Konrad 2005), while Melhuus and Howell (this volume) provide an intriguing example of a 'primitive form of artificial insemination' in 1902, and see Stolcke (1986) for commentary on the use of artificial insemination in 1799 in England and 1804 in France.
7. Like other culturally competent actors, anthropologists 'know' what belongs to the domain of biology.
8. Of interest here is Steven Rose's comment that the term 'biology' as a science has 'usurped its subject. So "biological" becomes the antonym not for "sociological" but for "social"' (Rose 1998: 5).
9. The current political regime in North America infamously categorised old and new Europe according to levels of agreement and compliance with its agenda; while from the perspective of the EU, Lithuania and Hungary, for example, are 'new' – each revealing the artifice of newness.
10. Responses to Schneider are rarely neutral. Parkin avers that he replaced Lévi-Strauss as 'the new kinship guru' (Parkin and Stone 2004: 18), and Kuper (1999) that he was a 'maverick'.
11. Schneider's work has been usefully located within broader shifts of interest in anthropology from function to meaning (Carsten 2004: 18) and from objectivist to reflexive approaches (Franklin and McKinnon 2001: 3).
12. From a Portuguese perspective, Mary Bouquet has argued that what is considered Western in terms of kinship is peculiarly British (1993). My own interest has been in what gets defined as 'British' kinship and how far analytical models are isomorphic with ethnography. Nonetheless, the project on which we report here flags a kinship of bureaucracy that is shared across a wide range of European contexts.
13. What I have called elsewhere, with tongue firmly in cheek, 'Euro-kin' (Edwards 2006).
14. We should also note here the strikingly different relationships that European publics appear to have with their governments: from the relatively acquiescent view of 'the state' and a confidence in the ability of government to govern in Norway, to vociferous critique of government and its agents in Spain and, perhaps, to an even greater degree in the UK.
15. The PUG project also included and was informed by research with black and mixed-heritage families in England (see Tyler 2005, 2007)
16. Franklin and McKinnon (2001) remind us that there had also been significant interventions from feminist perspectives including Gayle Rubin's (1975) prescient comments on the 'Eurocentrism of biologistic thinking'; and they

point to MacCormack and Strathern's (1980) edited collection which collates and develops anthropological debate since the 1960s on the status of 'natural facts'.
17. According to Schneider, shared 'biogenetic' substance and 'diffuse, enduring solidarity' were defining features of American kinship, which is 'primarily based upon European conceptions of the biological nature of human relationships (Ottenheimer 2001: 120). But both the biology to which he refers and his melding of biology and genetics require further attention.
18. Commercial surrogacy is not permitted across Europe and see Ragoné (2000) for an increasing preference for gestational surrogacy over 'traditional surrogacy' (where the surrogate mother is genetically linked to the ensuing child via her ova) in the US.
19. And see contributors to Edwards et al. (2007) and Edwards et al. (2008).
20. Developments in genetic medicine and the increasing use of genetic testing, for example, deploy biogenetic definitions of personhood and relatedness. They provoke an explicitness about who is genetically related to whom – not least because of the implications of the heritability of disease and disorder. Kaja Finkler, amongst others, argues that, with an increasing emphasis on genetic origins, diagnosis and therapy for certain medical disorders, a geneticisation of bodies, disease and relationships is occurring. She also refers to this as 'the medicalisation of family and kinship' (Finkler 2001).
21. Franklin, citing Haraway (1997), draw our attention to the way in which 'biology can make itself strange as quickly as any of its critics' (Franklin 2001: 320).
22. Strathern identifies three 'duplexes' that mark Euro-American kinship: 'connection/disconnection', 'conceptual/interpersonal' and 'a highly developed contrast between relations already in existence and those that must be deliberately created' (Strathern 2005: 8).
23. To borrow from Hemingway on Paris.
24. In contrast, for Nowotny and colleagues, science and society have ceased to operate as separate domains: they 'co-mingle' and are 'co-evolutionary' (Nowotny et al. 2001).
25. This exemplifies different approaches to kinship within PUG. It might crudely be described as the difference between French and Anglo-American tradition, which is not to suggest they 'belong' to French, British or North American scholarship but that they are shorthand for different theoretical and historical trajectories. To simplify and run the risk of stereotyping, one approach (let's call it post-structural or post-Lévi-Straussian) draws on a time-honoured practice of using language as a model for culture. Its central task is to reveal the logic in a cognitive or ideational system. From this perspective, the 'natural', physiological or biological 'facts' can be bracketed and the focus is on the syntagmatic relations between concepts. For Lévi-Strauss the genetic code and the linguistic code present the same characteristics and function in the same way. Another approach (let's call it post-constructivist or post-Schneiderian) starts with the premise that 'natural facts' are culturally produced, promoted and valued. Kinship from this perspective comprises a bunch of heterogeneous elements and the context (and intention) determines which will be deployed and brought to the fore in a particular instance. The emphasis here is on how kinship is 'done'.
26. It is partisan, for example, for The President's Council on Bioethics (PCBE), in its 2002 report on human cloning, to state categorically that: 'societies around

the world have structured social and economic responsibilities around the relationship between generations established through sexual procreation, and have developed modes of child rearing, family responsibility, and kinship behaviour that revolve around the natural facts of begetting' (2002: 9).

27. Or, in Harold Scheffler's (1991) terms, kinship is universally a matter of genealogy but not biology. Scheffler demands we pay attention to emic ideas of sex and reproduction and argues that the mother-child genealogical connection is universal: raising the question of how we theorise a genealogical connection between a mother and child conceived using donated ova and born to a surrogate mother.

CHAPTER 1

KNOWING AND RELATING:
KINSHIP, ASSISTED REPRODUCTIVE
TECHNOLOGIES AND THE NEW GENETICS

Joan Bestard

Tout se passe au milieu, tout transite entre les deux, tout se fait par médiation, par traduction et par réseaux, mais cet emplacement n'existe pas, n'a pas lieu. C'est l'impensé, l'impensable des modernes. (Latour 1991: 57)

Introduction

Before beginning my ethnographic discussion, I would like to define what I understand by kinship and how we can relate it to the public understanding of new genetics from an analytical point of view. I consider kinship as a tool that enables the anthropologist to analyse the capacity of certain ideas about human nature and the transmission of its substances to build social relations. The advantage of this type of analytical tool is that it is neither in the domain of nature nor in the domain of culture, but rather between the two and making the intermediation a domain that is neither within nor without, that is, a set of networks of unrelated entities, such as a network linking gametes, donors, parents, names, localities, identities and properties (Edwards and Strathern 2000). The advantage of conceiving kinship in terms of networks is that it implies no determinism, such as the determinism of genes on behaviour or of culture on relationships. Instead of expressing the problematic of kinship in terms of two pure transcendences ('nature' and 'culture'), thinking of kinship in this way allows us to ethnographically approach the existence of networks in both domains. Instead of attempting to explain kinship as a mixture of pure transcendences, the activity of the intersection of kinship becomes the source from which the domains of nature and culture originate (Latour 1991). For Latour, the social is not a special domain of reality, but a principle of connection between heterogeneous entities (2005: 13). In this way, the analytical pathway of kinship moves away from modernist ideologies that mix domains and attribute determinism to one (as the ideology of genetic essentialism does), and instead allows me to place ideas about human nature and entities coming from the technologies of reproduction within the formation of relationships.

As far as 'the public understanding of genetics' is concerned, I refer neither to the general public nor to a lay public as opposed to experts. I mean a particular ethnographically sited public, namely, couples wanting to have children through techniques of assisted reproduction (Bestard et al. 2003). By 'public understanding', I refer to what is understood in anthropology as culture, that is, the capacity to establish meaningful relationships between different domains of social life. It has more to do with the substantive rationality than with the formal rationality of the debate emerging from government advisory commissions (Evans 2002).

By 'new genetics', I mean the new knowledge stemming from the recent mapping of the human genome. This knowledge has opened up new possibilities for predicting and treating disease and genetic disorder. It has also opened up new ways to relate genes and human behaviour and new means of understanding human nature and society. It crosses the boundaries of two domains (subjects and objects) that have been separated in modernity. With the arrival of new hybrid entities coming from the new genetics, it is difficult to hold fast the modernist opposition between nature and culture. The 'natural' and the 'social' are no longer to be seen as ontologically different (Rheinberger 2000). The huge and complex organisation of the human genome can be compared with the complexity that anthropologists have discovered in society and cultural life. The complexity of kinship systems with only a few recombinant elements but hugely diverse meanings in different societies can be compared with the simple elements but complex organisation of the human genome. As François Jacob (1972) remarked, nature works to create diversity by means of unlimited combination of bits and pieces, namely, the four bases of DNA. New networks can be revealed between reproductive materials coming from laboratories, genes and the appropriation of them by people using assisted reproductive technologies (ART) in order to create new kinship relationships.

New reproductive technologies have to do with procreation and also with kinship, and my aim is to analyse how, in the context of assisted reproduction, kinship can be used to give meaning to a gamete's genetic endowment. Focusing on gamete donation, I address two questions. First, what is understood by a gamete? And second, what other materialities is it related to? My starting point is the methodological assumption that an object becomes meaningful in its relationship to other entities. Public understanding of scientific issues is not based on the content of the issue itself, but rather on the relationships it has with other heterogeneous entities. I understand kinship as a matrix that allows us to understand some of these matters by relating them to other unrelated entities, for instance, a network linking a gamete, a woman who is an egg donor, a legal mother, a name, a town and an identity. Thus placed, a gamete becomes one element in a network of relations. It is one element in a network of meaningful relationships and not only the recognition of a substance with a genetic endowment. Kinship knowledge is not the recognition of the facts of nature, but a tool to set up relations between divergent domains of life. It does not directly reflect the facts of nature, but relates what is 'given' and what is 'made' in social life.

The Ethnographic Meaning of a Gamete

The ethnographic question I wish to raise is simply, what is meant by a gamete? And, in particular, what is meant by an oocyte?

Berta is a woman from a town in the south of Spain. Every year she travels to Catalonia for a period of six or seven months in order to undergo infertility treatment and specifically a process of in vitro fertilisation (IVF). She and her husband take temporary jobs in the Costa Brava in the service sector. When we met her, Berta was working in the laundry of a hotel. Her husband had a temporary job as labourer in the construction industry. The rest of the year they have temporary jobs in agriculture in their village in southern Spain. Doctors had suggested that Berta should resort to oocyte donation. Despite the fact that gamete donation is anonymous in Spanish law, Berta was asked to look for a donor from whom she would receive the gametes. Because of the shortage of egg donors, this request is normal procedure in assisted reproduction clinics in Spain. The donor she brings to the clinic is meant to give her gametes to another anonymous woman and in exchange she will receive oocytes from another anonymous donor. Berta refuses to look for a donor on the grounds that she comes from a small town. Indeed, the closer a town comes to forming a community the stronger the feeling that everyone knows each other and is related to each other. This identity of mutual acquaintance comes precisely from the fact that residents were all born there and brought up together. Acquaintance, upbringing and kinship become one and the same thing. Referring to the possibility of finding a donor, our informant said:

> Maybe I am wrong, but what happens is ... if I look for a woman ... and besides if I look for her here [in Barcelona], they may not know about it in my town ... But if I looked for a woman in my town, because it is a small town, they would forever be saying ... that my child, for instance, is not mine. Maybe I'm too conscious of what people would say. But if I came here and I was told: 'Look, if you like ... I will give them to you, or if you like I could ... ', maybe I would. But having to look for a woman myself, no ... and besides, knowing, for instance, what they say that the one I find ... won't be the ones that they'll give me.

Berta argues that, if the egg donation is not anonymous, the donor could be considered the mother. Her town, where she was born and brought up, would immediately recognise the donor by just looking at the child and would therefore establish a relationship of descent, since in kinship a biological relationship is also a social relationship and a relationship of belonging is made via the model of concrete recognition of the kinship. In this case, only by remaining anonymous can the kinship relationship and the genetic relationship without social recognition be kept separate. Berta refuses to know the donor because this knowledge has consequences about her identity as mother. As Marilyn Strathern remarks, kinship knowledge is a form of constitutive rule: 'once known [it] can not be laid aside' (1999: 79). Berta exercises her right not to know by looking for an anonymous donor. Note also that she has in mind a hypothetical donor who is not from her hometown, where everyone knows each other and is related to each other. She has in mind someone from the city, another type of social conglomeration, where personal acquaintance between each of its members is impossible and which thus offers the anonymity she seeks. Our informant seeks a donation outside the actual relations of mutual acquaintances which, for her, are what kinship is. If the donation makes it possible to establish kinship it must be at a different level of knowledge from the relation with the donor of her village, that is, relations between individual persons. She is looking for an abstract sociality, that is, an anonymous and nameless relation (Konrad 2005). That is why she associates the egg donation with the anonymity of the city, and not with the face-to-face community of her town. If it became known in her town, people would say the child was not hers. Gamete donation implies identity, and donation is an alienation of something that carries with it the identity of the donor. In contrast, in the city identity remains anonymous and social relations are abstract. That is why she thinks it is easier to find an abstract, anonymous and nameless donor in the city. Thus she comes closer to goods circulating freely on the market than to donation where a particular relationship is established between the donor and receiver through the gift. The debt of the gift is to an anonymous donor, not to an individual person from her hometown, even if kinship is a way to establish relations outside market commodities.

The paradox in Berta's narrative is how to understand the relationship stemming from a donation and how another woman's gamete can become an element in her own descent. Here I would like to emphasise the point that an issue concerning genetics can lead to a series of associations between heterogeneous entities – a gamete, a donation, the town, the city, an identity and a property. How does the relation between a gamete and a given person manage to become the relation between the receptor and her offspring? For Berta, the donation from a woman in her hometown would suppose identification between the person and the object donated. That is why, for her, the anonymity of the city is a resource with which she can think about this transformation.

Ben Amar and Rahisa, a Moroccan couple living in Catalonia, repeat this association between the gamete and the donor. 'I think the child would be another person's,' says Ben Amar, and he insists on the relationship between offspring and 'blood'. 'Surely [I want] the child, but from my own blood, I insist, from my *own blood*.' He considers the association between offspring and one's own blood, and a donation and the relationship with another person, as a cultural relationship: 'It would become engraved on my brain that this child was not mine.' It is as if he would not be able to recognise himself in a possible offspring conceived through a donated gamete. Genetic discontinuity requires a reconsideration of the continuity of descent expressed in the idea of 'one's own blood'. When I refer to culture I do not refer to a system of meanings differentiating one ethnic group from another, but the relationships that are established through the possibility of donation: gametes related to a donor as opposed to blood, male descent and knowledge.

Esperança, who has recently given birth to a child thanks to ova donation, felt the rejection of a friend towards her child because 'she must have seen that my part was missing … It has been difficult for her to relate to my child'. Relating is culture's work, through which it opens windows that establish relationships between a gamete, the recipient and her offspring. By not being able to relate to the child immediately, Esperança's friend perceives two separate bodies and cannot establish a relationship because she cannot visualise the connection between mother and child. Offspring are perceived to be the result of the relationship between two people. 'It's a bit of each', said Isa, who, with two children from a former relationship, wanted to have a child with her new partner. If the link with the oocyte is not known, it is difficult to establish a relationship between mother and child. The anonymity of the donation brings about an immediate paradox. As Isa narrates her experience as recipient, she says that, 'since the genes are from an unknown source' and 'we don't know where the genes come from', you 'don't quite regard it as your own. I see it as foreign'. A gamete is also a relationship. It is not merely a biological substance making new individuals possible, but is located within the scope of kinship relations. Because it is relational, it has to do with the donor. In our research, the term 'genetic mother' was never mentioned, but, in the case of oocyte donations, the genes clearly come from another woman, and therefore from an unknown and perhaps unknowable relational chain. This gap in knowledge poses practical problems such as not knowing what to tell the paediatrician when he or she asks about family history illnesses, or not knowing what to say to the child in the future.

Idioms of Ownership: to Have One's Own Child

Thus far, I have dealt with one important aspect regarding the way kinship knowledge is organised. It is a relationship that looks back to the past. Memories, stories of the past and inheritances are all elements linked with the past. People are our relatives because we relate them to a common ancestor. Nevertheless, kinship also has to do with the present and the future. Relatedness not only arises from the past, but is also built in the present and looks towards the future (Bestard 1998). Descent not only implies ancestors, but also descendants. In this case, descent is personally constructed in that it is clearly desired and planned. This element of agency in kinship is very much present in the context of assisted reproductive technologies (ART). After all, it involves men and women who desire a child. That is, they have imagined their offspring and seek, in ART, the possibility of making their 'dream for a child' come true. In this context, a 'donated gamete' does not mean a connection in the present with another person, but the possibility of a new relationship in the future. 'I then found myself pregnant,' says the woman who had doubts about the identity of the embryo that results from a donated ova. At the moment of finding herself pregnant she establishes a relationship with her future child. From here on, connections are made into the future, that is, the model of establishing kinship creates links between various entities: gametes, pregnancy, child-rearing, ownership and identity.

This element of agency in the establishment of relationships is well expressed by Esperança who keeps a diary in the form of a letter to her future child before starting an IVF cycle. First, the offspring is conceived in the mind and then the desire is materialised in the body. The diary begins like this:

> Dear child,
> I have wanted you for so long that now it is difficult to write thinking of you as a reality, though we are still far from that moment ... Maybe I should introduce myself first: if everything goes right, I'll be your [*el teu o el vostre*] (maybe there will be more than one of you) mother. Today it still seems difficult – though possible – that someone should name me like this, but then, I want it so badly! ... Actually, I've had this desire to be a mother inside me for so long that I cannot recall the first time I felt it ... Now in a way you are already here among us, as a thought, as a construction of the future.

This diary becomes a highly reflexive process of how to establish new kinship relations. It constitutes a reflexive process, which is also very characteristic of people entering into cycles of assisted reproduction, as they must relate and make the reproductive substances that the clinic manipulates in the laboratory meaningful, out of the context of the relations that give meaning to the body and its reproductive substances. Faced with oocyte donation, Esperança reflects in her diary on how to explain the donation to her friends:

> I debated in my mind for some days whether to tell everyone or just my closest friends, those who could better understand that you would be born in my belly, but with another woman's genetic endowment. It is true I debated whether to tell them or not because it was also difficult for me to accept it myself. I had been secretly thinking of you for so long that I had begun to project my wishes; for instance, that you would inherit my nose,

which is a distinguishing mark of our family, that you could have my father's blue eyes (your grandfather, whom you will never meet). I was also afraid that your father could one day argue that you were genetically his child in order to take you away from me.

Faced with a donation and a future child having 'the genetic endowment of another woman', she is forced to question different forms of relationship, family identity and belonging. With a bit of nostalgia for continuity with the past, Esperança thinks her child will not have that nose so characteristic of her family, or her father's eyes. She also thinks this discontinuity will make it possible for her child not to 'inherit certain things I don't like at all of my family'. Notice that family inheritance is totally amoral, you inherit for good and bad. Any discontinuity opens, therefore, the possibility of a greater diversity and variability in the future. Nevertheless, genetic continuity is a powerful tool when one thinks about belonging. She is torn between immediate belonging, which makes genetic continuity possible (homologous to genealogical continuity): 'The first thing I thought', she says, 'was that it will be his, not mine.' Her husband can establish a genetic continuity, but she has to repair this discontinuity. Her husband, a Latin American emigrant of Spanish origin, told me the first time we met that his family in Latin America was very happy about the new baby because it would be the first grandchild born in Spain after three generations. Continuity is genetic and territorial. For him, the *ius sanguinis* of citizenship law has met again with *ius soli*, after a three-generation gap. Esperança, however, looks at it from a different angle: how will the child become 'mine'? In other words, how will she establish continuity between present and future? When her child was born, she explained – not without irony – that people visiting them, and without knowing about the egg donation, were talking of the likeness between her and the child. They were making connections of likeness across her family lines. She concluded by saying how important pregnancy is to identify with a child: pregnancy blurs biological milieu and genetic endowment. She has been pregnant, given birth and fed her child. Across these very biological and cultural actions she has passed on substances of her body and has identified herself with the child. Therefore the child resembles her and she thinks in terms of continuity.

A series of metaphors exists in kinship that make this connection possible – metaphors that often arise in ethnographic contexts of assisted reproduction when the topic of what it means to have a child comes up, even when referring to offspring stemming from one's own gametes. Children (*'neixen i es crien'*) 'are born and bred', 'we have them and we make them' (*es tenen i es crien*), 'they are not only children, but they become children' (*els fills no sòn, es fan*) are common expressions. I do not consider these metaphors to mean that nature (born) gives way to culture (bred), but they refer to the interactive element of kinship relationships. Kinship, as we have seen, belongs neither to the domain of nature nor to that of culture, but it is between the two. It makes intermediation a domain of its own neither within nor without, but rather the place of networks linking up different entities.

Although kinship often uses the language of natural substances – gametes, genes, blood – it refers to relationships between people and it links heterogeneous entities (not only gametes with genes, but gametes with identities, that is, bodies and substances with properties).

These relationships of belonging and identity end up relativising the language of natural substances. In the process of appropriating offspring and creating identity, as Esperança says, 'one ends up thinking that the genetic endowment is not all that determining': family identity is not reduced to a set of genes, but is a relational element. The advantage of conceiving kinship in terms of networks is that it does not imply determinism of network links. Instead, property appears as an interactive process. As Esperança says:

> I'll carry the child nine months in my womb, how could he/she not be mine? You have carried it inside you, you have nourished it, fed it ... you have passed your feelings, thoughts, emotions on to him/her during these nine months, you will give birth to him/her, ... well, I do not know whose this child can be if it is not mine. I know, the genetic endowment ... in the end it's relativised, isn't it?

The relationship implies an appropriation and therefore a process in which you manage to get 'a child of your own'. Property here does not mean an exclusive right between two people, or between a person and a gamete, or the reification of an element (genes, for instance) that determines appropriation. It is rather a relationship that links a new object of science with new identities. Paraphrasing Strathern (1999: 161), I would say that the object of Esperança's knowledge – the donated gamete – has been appropriated in a new way and her intention for using it is the indicator of her creativity and her capacity to anticipate her future as mother.

Discussion

I would like to touch on the idea of the progressive geneticisation of human behaviours and of the family that has made new genetics possible (Finkler 2000, 2001). There is of course a public discourse – of the media, basically – that tends to reduce the person to a set of genes and to convert genes into the determining factor not only of physical ailments, but also of 'social evils'. This considered, it has been pointed out that with the arrival of new genetics a progressive geneticisation of the concept of human nature occurs, with a consequent determinism attributed to genes, which in turn not only offers the possibility of preventing illness, but also behaviour traits – a process by which the human being is reduced to a bunch of genes. Critics call it 'genetic essentialism'; that is, the reduction of a person to inherited qualities that influence the course of his or her life. This ideology relates individual attributes to social problems to the point that these can be dealt with in the field of clinical genetics. As a result, a person's identity is better defined in biological terms than in social terms. The relational viewpoint disappears from the identity discourse and is reduced to a set of inherited characters.

The idea of progressive geneticisation does not seem to fit properly the ethnographic facts we have just presented, where genes are seen in the context of assisted reproduction. Esperança admitted that she had always thought that 'genetics leaves a mark', but faced with the 'facts of assisted reproduction' and thinking about them in the context of basic kinship relationships, she ended up 'relativising genes'. In other words, she sees them within a network of relationships of heterogeneous entities. In her diary she has created a new moral landscape (Pálsson and Hardardóttir 2002) to situate gamete donation. She uses the 'flexible choreography' (Thomson 2001) of the complex interplay of kinship knowledge.

In this moral landscape, the use of metaphors such as 'blood' or 'genes' can sound deterministic, but they can also be very flexible. The flexibility of these metaphors arises when there is no marked distinction between the domains of nature and culture, and heterogeneous entities are mobilised – gametes, information, donation, conception, maternity, chid-rearing, ownership, and so on. In this case, identities are formed through the relationships between these elements. It is not a rigid pattern. A child, as we have seen, is born and bred. Both activities are closely linked with kinship; they do not necessarily imply a move from nature to culture. A mother who has gestated her child from a donated gamete can say the child is 'hers'. Appropriation takes place during gestation and rearing, that is, as part of parentship, and this belongs to the domain of nature as well as culture. If this is true, neither nature nor culture is essentialised, but they rather become metaphors for thinking and imagining relatedness. The fact that a child resembles his/her parents does not necessarily imply genetic determinism, but a relationship that is formed through nature in constant interaction. These ideas do not come from public discourses on science, but rather from fieldwork experience regarding kinship relationships. In my previous fieldwork carried out in Formentera, people said that a child resembled the godparent (Bestard 1991). This did not contradict the physical resemblance the child had with its parents, or the fact that the child inherits moral and physical characters from the house it belongs to.

We must be aware that the process of establishing links through heterogeneous entities is more complex than the concepts of either biologisation or geneticisation of social relationships suggest. It is much more indeterminate; it is mediation between heterogeneous elements and it can colonise different areas of social life without necessarily referring to biology or to culture in the strict sense of the terms. It operates within the area from which ideas related to transmitted substances and relationships arise – an undefined area where things, traits, attributes are naturalised and culturalised at the same time.

The stories of our informants regarding genetics and heredity are much more complex and contradictory than what the critics of the geneticisation process generally claim. I would say they are as complex as the theoretical discourse of biology, anthropology and genetics. In their conversation we can detect points of view that define different ways of relating heterogeneous elements. Whereas from one point of view numerous aspects of human behaviour are reduced to the action of specific genes, from another perspective the role of interaction is central. The matrix of this complex issue can be found in cultural ideas of kinship: that is, in the place where people attribute meaning to biological substances in the construction of social relationships, and in the capacity that networks of kinship have to change points of view.

This leads us to the way culture functions in anthropology and how to analyse 'public understanding'. Culture is not the recognition of the facts of nature, as kinship was thought to be in earlier anthropological kinship studies. It is essentially a way to analyse people's assumptions regarding the meaning and value they give to certain behaviour (Strathern 1997b: 41). For example, 'to be of the same blood' is an aspect of culture which means that a common biological substance runs through the veins of all our relatives. However this statement is imprecise; it cannot be interpreted literally. It does not necessarily follow that the members of a given family share common genes. As we have seen, reducing kinship to genetics becomes absurd and paradoxical in certain contexts of assisted reproduction.

Culture opens the way not only to assumptions, but also to the implications of these assumptions. It deals not only with how values are mobilised, but also with how chains of ideas in complex areas of social life are constructed. For example, the values that the techniques of assisted reproduction mobilise lead to a reassessment of the role biology plays in establishing social links. Ideas always function in the context of other ideas. Contexts form semantic domains that separate ideas and at the same time connect them. Finally, culture leads to reflexivity (Strathern 1997b: 44). It is not only the analysis of people's assumptions regarding certain facets of social life, but the analytical assumptions we use to make our analysis. David Schneider, in his critique of kinship studies, observed that what anthropologists understood by kinship was linked to a very specific representation of knowledge. For Schneider, 'The Euro-American notion of knowledge depended on the proposition that knowledge is *discovered*, not invented, and that knowledge comes when the "facts" of nature, which are hidden from us mostly, are finally revealed' (Schneider 1995: 222). In earlier kinship studies, there was a reference to a biological space that was characterised as the hidden nature to be discovered. In this sense kinship could be reduced to newly discovered scientific facts of reproduction. This naturalistic representation of knowledge and kinship has a strong appeal, even if ethnography demonstrates that kinship is a way to establish relations between heterogeneous entities and not a social relation to be reduced to the discovered facts of nature.

CHAPTER 2

IMAGINING ASSISTED REPRODUCTIVE TECHNOLOGIES: FAMILY, KINSHIP AND 'LOCAL THINKING' IN LITHUANIA

Auksuolė Čepaitienė

Concerns with biogenetic technologies have recently become a topic of public interest in Lithuania. New efforts to create a legal context for biomedical research and assisted reproduction in Lithuania in the late 1990s stimulated an openness in dealing with themes which were previously under the shadow of a respect for science during the Soviet era. It turned out that looking at assisted reproductive technologies (ART) as social and cultural facts was a new experience for many Lithuanians. This chapter examines the way in which Lithuanians construct and contextualise their ideas about ART. It points to the questions of how people claim their identities and affiliations and what ideas they employ in negotiating their sense of belonging. But mainly the chapter draws on local thinking about family and kinship, which emerges in the challenges that scientific developments present.[1] In elucidating this, first I shall briefly describe my theoretical standpoint and introduce the ethnographic setting. Then, I shall turn to Lithuanian people's ideas on ART, family and kinship by following the way in which they narrate their understandings by moving from concrete answers to general considerations.

Theorising ART and Kinship

Many recent anthropological works have argued that discussion on ART provides a critical account for new kinship studies (e.g. Peletz 1991; Strathern 1992a, 1992b; Edwards et al. 1993; Ragoné 1994; Holy 1996;

Edwards 1999; Franklin 2001; Bestard 2004a; Carsten 2004; Parkin, and Stone 2004; Orobitg, and Salazar 2005). In my study I consider the categories of kinship and of community as theoretical and methodological positions of a priori and analytical instruments that facilitate the development of a space for cross-cultural approaches. Starting from kinship and community this study inevitably turns to local thinking. I understand local thinking to mean, first of all, the knowledge an anthropologist gets from local people, that is from a particular ethnographic site defined through social, geographical, and temporal dimensions – the time of the community under research. But I also see local thinking as a way of analysing the question in a particular socially and culturally interrelated setting. The latter aspect is always present as 'the shapes of knowledge are always ineluctably local, indivisible from their instruments and their encasements' (Geertz 1983: 4). This means that discourses of ART and kinship fostered together 'assist' one another (Edwards 2000) and the anthropological images produced in this way are closer to social reality, however partial (Clifford 1986), than the universal, holistic and totalitarian overview.

Next to interconnected issues of ART and kinship lies the question of personhood and identity which is no less significant for ART and for kinship studies of today (Strathern 1992a, 1997a; Edwards 1999, 2005; Carsten 2004). It is David Schneider who in the late 1960s liberated a person from kinship ties (1968, 1984, 1996). He places the person in a central position by looking 'at the relative as a person and at the person as a relative' and claiming that the person – a relative – is a cultural unit, 'just as family, the company, the city and the country (the nation) are' (Schneider 1968: 57). Marilyn Strathern, emphasising the choice and individual complexity of persons, goes further. Her assumption that individual persons are somehow prior to the relationship (Strathern 1992a: 53) is crucial for anthropological understanding of kinship, where the person might be recognised as independent of kin relationships, as a loop or apex in the kin network (Astuti 2000) or as an agent identified through a variety of 'kinning' strategies (Carsten 1995a, 2000b; Howell 2003).

The issue of personhood and identity, despite the fact that it has questioned the 'respectful' academic position of kinship (Howell and Melhuus 1993), made an impulse for new methodological directions, and reinforced the extension of ethnographic research in the late 1970s and early 1980s (Strathern 1981; Cohen 1982; Boholm 1983; Bestard 1991; Segalen 1991). As Edwards says: 'It has been the issues of identity and belonging and local conceptualisation of boundaries which have emerged as theoretically significant in recent ethnography ... Identity and belonging to both people and places, are aspects of persons, which mobilise and are mobilised by kinship thinking' (2000: 26). Consideration of identity is an urgent topic of many ethnographic studies of the post-Soviet world, including Lithuania. Evidently, the discourses and representations of 'self' and belonging after the fall of the Soviet Union become significant factors in the transformation of societies (Skultans

1998; Wanner 1998; Berdahl 1999; Verdery 1999; Čepaitienė 2004; Rausing 2004). Representations of 'self' and belonging, I suggest, reproduce also a space for 'local thinking'.

In my study I take the categories of identity and personhood together with those of community and kinship to the ethnography of Lithuanian society. It is a 'travel' (Hastrup and Hervik 1994) where the individual encountered is both an active agent and a cultural universe (Strathern 1992a; Sökefeld 1999) full of and framed by his/her personal experiences and lifestyles, world views and ideological considerations, stages of life and ageing (Astuti 2000), gendered physical and social considerations of being and reproducing, and many other large and small things that are significantly related in kaleidoscopic ways. I expect the discourses of identity, personhood and belonging to act as instrumental notions through which critical accounts on thinking about ART and kinship can be provided.

The Place and the People: the Town of Kuršėnai

In the autumn of 2002 my colleague Darius Daukšas and I went to Kuršėnai, a small town in western Lithuania located close to the seat of the administrative district Šiauliai. It was my second visit there; the first had been in 1999. Our intention was to investigate people's thinking about ART in the way Edwards had done in Alltown (1993, 1998, 1999, 2000, 2002).[2] Kuršėnai is to some extent comparable to Alltown, though they have different economic histories. Today it has about 15,800 residents, but before the Second World War Kuršėnai was a town with a population of between 3,000 and 4,000. It began to grow at the end of the 1930s with pottery crafts, and a sugar factory and a brick factory were established in the interwar period. These lines of production were the main industries during the Soviet period and their capacities significantly increased with the brick factory, for example, expanding into the production of building materials. However, when we arrived in 2002, the sugar factory was operating only in the autumn and winter and the building materials factory was closed.

Kuršėnai is a fairly homogeneous community of ethnic Lithuanians (about 90 per cent), the remainder being mainly ethnic Russians, Latvians and Poles. Before the Second World War there was a large Jewish community in the town, members of which were mainly engaged in trading activities and business while the ethnic Lithuanians were involved with the local administration, the state educational sphere and the Catholic Church. Historically, there had always been a manor estate the owner of which was Polish. However, the Second World War and post-war events resulted in the loss of the majority of former citizens in disastrous ways. The present-day community of Kuršėnai is comprised of people who settled in the town, mainly after the Second World War from the surrounding villages and more distant areas. Although there are some four- and five-storyed Soviet-style apartment blocks in the town, many people live in private houses. Each house has a garden and plenty of space for growing flowers and vegetables and for keeping domestic animals. The everyday life of residents is anchored in a closed family circle, with a few relatives, friends and neighbours, co-workers and friends. Undoubtedly, the neighbourhood is significant in the functioning of the social space, where, as one interviewee said, 'everybody knows everything about everybody'. The relationship between neighbours is represented in small exchanges related to daily matters, or sharing information 'over the fence'. Emphasising this, I nonetheless speak about the small 'society' of the town of Kuršėnai as structured into segmented social worlds instead of 'a tightly-knit community' (Edwards and Strathern 2000: 151) where 'community space as a whole is generally a shared experience' (Pocius 1991: 272).

We went to the field with Schneider in mind. He said that 'in a very fundamental sense the anthropologist is like a child who must be socialised' (Schneider 1968: 9), and that 'learning the culture is just like learning the language' (1968: 10). The ethnographic reality Darius and I met with in Kuršėnai is the interactive space of thoughts, ideas, narratives and images rather than social experiences that are overt in society (see Barth 2002). We considered the aspects of narrating, naming and discourse of particular significance for our study (Schneider 1968; Boholm 1983; Hill and Mannheim 1992; Ricoeur 2000; Bourdieu 2002). However, we realised that 'language events' are but a fraction of what constitutes the 'material' (Hastrup and Hervik 1994). We treat our relationship with interviewees to be that of fellow participants who would help clarify Lithuanian thinking about ART (see Boholm 1983; Hastrup 1996; Edwards 2002). Moreover, we ourselves as well as the wider project in which we were embedded were also significant participants in the interaction, affecting people's understanding and knowledge, and diminishing the cultural neutrality of the situation (see Turner 2000).

Our study in Kuršėnai is mainly based on immediate interviews and conversations. We conducted semi-structured interviews with forty-nine people and asked the opinion of twenty-nine students from the senior class of a secondary school. We took into account the totality of our experiences, including people's enthusiasms and silences as well as their refusals to speak with us and their ways of politely evading the conversation. Our ethnographic enquiry is, to some extent, gendered in the sense that Darius spoke mostly with men, and I with women. Among our interviewees there are middle-aged and elderly couples, newly-weds, married and divorced women and men and grandmothers living with their children and grandchildren; there are teachers, workers at the sugar factory and agriculture company, shop assistants, unemployed people, established residents and newcomers. There are those who emphasised that they are no longer concerned with the issues of ART because they are past childbearing age, or already had children, and those who reported that they supported childless couples who are thinking about using ART, as well as those who were definitely against ART. But in general they are all part of the same community and society of which we are also members.

The Discourse on ART and What Comes Next

All the interviewees knew about ART. They acquired most of their information from television, newspapers, women's journals, radio broadcasts and lessons at school. Our ethnographic enquiry was held at a time when drafted legislation for the law on assisted reproduction was approved by the Seimas of the Republic of Lithuania (Parliament). Some people, in particular women, had already discussed it in smaller, intimate circles of friends. It seems that the question of ART enters into the conversation of women more naturally than that of men, although we discovered that it is of serious concern to men also.

ART is not a subject of ordinary everyday chats. Sometimes the opinions of people are framed in the style of 'taking sides' (Schlee 2004), or speakers circle around the topic with superficial talk, including sexual innuendo. To talk about ART with or without prejudice also labels the person as being either modern and liberal or traditional and old-fashioned. We observed, however, that, in all cases where discussion went beyond the superficial, it inevitably became serious and more complicated, full of doubts and emphasis, which were similar in all conversations.

People began their narratives on ART by looking at ART as a particular kind of technology – a scientifically constructed and medically performed alternative to natural procreation.[3] Interviewees then placed this general and abstract idea within imagined but concrete, personally familiar and analogous situations: within actual or potential experience. It is this intersection between the general and the personal, the abstract and the concrete, at which cultural beliefs are arranged and moral considerations are formulated.

To generalise, Kuršėnai residents' narratives about ART revolve around the following themes: infertility and the wish to have a child; scientific innovation, medical help and test-tube stories; adoption and the child as the genetic product of both partners; the unknown donor and the 'outsider' entering the family; 'blood' connections and paternity; aspects of 'artificial' and 'natural'; surrogacy, motherhood and sperm banks; spirituality and world view. But the main themes that underlie all these ideas are those of family (*šeima*) and conjugality (see Hirsch 1993).

In these stories no mention is made of kinship (*giminystė*). When we asked interviewees about the relationship between ART and kinship, they denied it categorically, saying that it is neither a question of relatives nor of kin. There is the difference between the Lithuanian words *giminystė/giminė* and *šeima*.[4] *Giminystė* (kinship) denotes the relationship of being a kinsperson and includes an extended group of kinsmen – *giminė* (family, kin and relatives), while *šeima* (family) means a social group consisting of parents and children, including relatives or the other people who live together and share common activities: in this sense it is closer to household.

According to interviewees, kinship is thought to disturb the privacy of the family and intimacy of procreation. Rasa Paukštytė (1999) has shown that in Lithuanian village life the woman during the period of pregnancy gradually leaves public life in the community and towards the end she stays entirely at home, with a midwife and sometimes a husband or other family member participating in the delivery. She returns to public life with the newborn child after a period of time after the birth. Traditionally the pregnancy and birth are surrounded by shadows, silence and secrecy (see Thiessen 1999: 193), and the community – neighbours and kinsmen – retreat. The interviewees in Kuršėnai deal with ART in the same manner. They act as the moral gatekeepers of an intimate sphere of the family, placing ART and procreation within the relationship of the husband and wife. ART and medical doctors are expected to participate in the event by providing medical assistance, but maintaining social neutrality. Nevertheless, the question of ART is not screened out: the interviewees pay attention to it.

The Family Where a Child Acts as 'Glue'

It is the desire of infertile couples to have a child that is the main axis of the stories told to us about ART. To Darius's question 'What is ART?' a forty-five year-old married man Alvydas, working in the local agricultural company, answers: 'Well ... Well, simply, if a woman can't get pregnant, if she wants children ... A family without children isn't [a family] ... There's no reason [for a family to be].' According to him and many others, a husband and wife are 'a family' and their relationship is established through marriage. They live together and 'have common interests'. Cohabiting together, being in close proximity to each other and experiencing the myriad of daily exchanges (Simpson 1998: 7), they establish a connection in time which is defined through everyday discourse, mutual understanding and togetherness. Their experience of a multitude of relationships results in them becoming part of one another, and this might be a durable tie. As a young unmarried woman explained: 'Spouses living in a stable family somehow become identical and similar to each other in respect of behaviour and even appearance.'

But, as Alvydas says, the family needs a 'reason (*argumentas*)' for existing. According to him, a husband and wife are also 'two strangers living together', who could easily split and revert into two non-related parts. They might begin to disintegrate and split, and childlessness or infertility could be a significant factor in this. Interviewees see infertility as a serious and 'natural' reason for divorce. Although they talk of procreation as occurring between both a husband and wife, they attribute infertility to one spouse or the other. This is a different way of looking at infertility from that in infertility clinics studied by Cussins, where the patient in treatment is not the individual person, but rather the infertile couple, with women's body parts standing in for the couple (Cussins1998: 69). The interviewees in Kuršėnai personalise infertility, although it is not always stigmatised. Alongside stories about sexual freedom being a cause of infertility, or it being the 'fault' of the woman or the man, there are stories about the Chernobyl nuclear catastrophe and its effect on men's infertility, and the fact that a person might be born infertile. Moreover, they think that infertility is not always identifiable through medical examination. Our interviewees report that sometimes there seems to be something mutually inadequate – that partners do not fit each other. Interviewees give examples of couples who, while living together, had no children but who had children after they had divorced and established a new family. Although infertile couples might live in harmony, the fact that one partner is infertile is an important reason why family ties 'split naturally (*savaime išsiskiria*)'.

The relationship between two individuals – the husband and wife – requires, then, a kind of fixture (Strathern 1992a; Edwards 1993; Ragoné 1994). And a child appears to be the 'reason' that motivates, justifies and fixes the relationship of husband and wife. Being the 'reason' for the family, the child becomes the 'glue' in the relationship between husband and wife (Simpson 1998). As Bob Simpson writes, 'reference to children as a kind of conjugal glue is one I have heard among divorced people who have re-married and for whom the arrival of a child is a powerful statement of authentication, legitimization and connection' (1998: 63). He has shown that the birth of children or the decision to become parents was the point at which couples decided to convert a cohabiting relationship into a conjugal relationship (1998: 63).

This is also the view of Elena, an older woman working in Kuršėnai children's hospital. Commenting on her positive consideration of ART she says: 'There's no reason to have ten, but one is a necessity. That child is a bond. If God won't bestow that gift, then at least there's this. There are those who take children from orphanages, but it's better to have one's own genes.' Her notion that 'a child is a bond' recalls the words of another woman, Ona, who was reluctant to express her negative opinion of ART because the fact of having children 'means life itself' for families. There, as well as in the narratives of other interviewees, the child is expected to participate in the social intertwining of 'inter-personal commitment, dependency and exchange' (Simpson 1998: x), and to mediate the existing relationship between a husband and a wife. It creates a prospect for their connection and draws on the future – the project – of family (Hirsch 1993: 78). Establishing a purpose to life it becomes a 'reason', a 'glue', a 'necessity' that 'means life itself'.

I would like to turn at this point to a closer look at how residents of Kuršėnai perceive the relationship between husband and wife in general. This appears to be the place where the question of kinship emerges, albeit in its absence.

In Between a Husband and a Wife

Although husband and wife are considered to be a family, the relationship is not seen as a kinship tie. Commenting on what kinship is, the majority of interviewees emphasise the specificity of the relationship between husband and wife and withdraw it from the category of kin relations. It is said that, although 'friends (*draugai*)', they are 'two strangers living together' who 'become like kin', or 'are closer than kin': 'closer than brothers and sisters' or 'the closest human beings'. But they 'do not become ... kin in a real, actual sense (*giminė tai aišku nepasidaro*)'.

I spoke with three young women: Dalia and Vilma are divorced and Lina is a newly wed. To my question 'Are they relatives?' referring to husband and wife, they all answer in chorus and with a laugh that they are not: 'we do not rank', 'recognise' and 'consider' a husband as a relative, and we 'do not want to have such relatives'. They use the social practice of divorce and its legally sanctioned possibility as an explanation for why husband and wife are not related as kin. Further conversation shows that Dalia still maintains a relationship with her ex-husband and his parents and her son stays with them. She says that children tie a husband and wife but nevertheless they remain strangers. According to Vilma the relationship between children and their father is a particular one. It extends into the future and does not depend on the fact of divorce. But it is not the same one that exists between her and her ex-husband: 'He is the father of my children, but for me he is not a relative [laugh].' She puts it with irony, 'today – kin, and tomorrow ... '. Kinship in her and the other women's mind is an enduring relationship without any prospect for split or cleavage, even when contacts are strained or severed.

Evidently kinship here is understood by the consideration of particular properties that exist prior to marriage. As Dalia tells it: a husband and wife, 'they were not relatives before the marriage, they did not become relatives after the marriage either'. This particular property is rooted in kin identity established through sameness of 'blood', which is absent in the relation between husband and wife. Listen to the opinion of a retired older woman, Janina.

> He [a husband] is practically not kin. A stranger [a laugh]. A good friend only. He is usually considered to be kin. But practically he is not. Although people usually maintain the kinship ties, and consider him to be kin, it is usually said that there is the kindred of the husband and the kindred of the wife. For children ... they [a husband and children] are real kin ... but for the wife [he is] ... with her [laugh] – well, it's only written down in the papers (*kągi, popierius surašo*). For children it becomes the same blood (*tas pats kraujas*).

The 'blood (*kraujas*)' as a conceptually significant icon of kinship draws a line of separation between husband and wife and acts as a criterion for categorising people into kin and non-kin. The 'blood' allocates them into those who are 'real (*tikroji*)' or 'natural (*natūrali*)' kin and those who are 'half kin (*pusiau giminės*)' or 'kin-like (*kaip giminės*)'. Operating as a symbolic sign under which people may be traced and recruited and as a way of connecting and disconnecting people, the 'blood' is perceived to be a durable and empowered image. It might be 'pure (*grynas*)' and 'purified (*išgrynintas*)', 'true (*tikras*)' and 'one's own (*savas*)', or 'mother's blood (*motinos kraujas*)' and 'father's blood (*tėvo kraujas*)'. However the ethnographic examples demonstrate its mobility and dynamism and refer to its conventionality (see Schneider 1968). 'Blood' might 'mix (*maišosi*)', 'fade (*išblunka*)', 'dilute (*skiedžiasi*)' and 'wash out (*išsiplauna*)', and it might 'call (*šaukiasi*)', 'attract (*traukia*)' or be given to the other. In one case it appears that one has a 'blood relation (*kraujo ryšys*)' and in another that the 'blood relation almost disappeared'. Various cultural and social items might 'interfere (*įsiterpti*)', be added or move together with 'blood': money, wealth, land, time, social standing, 'erudition', communication, kind-heartedness, character, politics, religion, law and knowledge.

The criterion of 'blood' that assists in drawing a boundary between husband and wife is also employed in Kuršėnai residents' stories as the matrimonial rule against incest (see Lévi-Strauss 1969; Porqueres i Gené 2000; and Porqueres i Gené and Wilgaux, this volume). Interviewees' explanations that they are not of the 'same blood' were usually elaborated by the statement that 'kin are not allowed to marry' and often with a laugh, which encoded both sexual intercourse between a husband and a wife, and its prohibition between kinsfolk called 'blood-mixing (*kraujomaiša*)'.

I suggest that the development of the themes of family and conjugality in the stories on ART activate the wider context of marriage and matrimonial rules and, finally, that of kinship. Enric Porqueres i Gené (2000), referring to Lévi-Strauss and Héritier, argues that marriage organises a particular understanding of kinship where kinsmen are identified by the sameness of 'blood', and bodily images appear as powerful representations. He also stresses that the idea of 'blood' kinship is not the primary one, but a result of matrimonial rules. I see this represented in my interviewees' thinking when they say that husband and wife are not kin, but kinship is established in their union.

Where Kinship Is Not a Family

It seems that the boundary between husband and wife, which is marked with 'blood', is stretching further between the social arrangements of family and kinship. This distinction might even be described using the idioms of 'social' and 'biological'. However, when the account shifts away from microscopic analysis of the relationship between husband and wife, the view becomes more sophisticated.

I recall the opinion of a young hairdresser, Kristina. Our conversation begins with an explanation of our research project and extends to assisted reproduction, her family and her son, who had epilepsy, and the cases of infertility among her friends. She tells me about her four brothers, sisters-in-law, parents, parents-in-law and her husband's sister, and says that they all communicate. Even though they live at considerable distances from one another, they often visit each other for no reason at all, or they come together on days of celebration, such as birthdays, Easter or marriage anniversaries. To my question 'What is kinship?', Kristina answers with confidence: 'It is clear to everyone.' She continues by listing parents, children, grandparents and grandchildren. Along with them she mentions the 'family'. But, when asked about whether husband and wife are kin, she presents a different perspective: 'They are not kin, yet they become part of the kindred group somehow. You know, a husband's kindred become the kin of the wife in time. They do not become relatives, but as close as such. But not kin in the real, actual sense'. She adds that it is impossible to become kin because of 'the genes' and explains that kinship is genes: 'Let's say, children – my children and the children of my husband's sister are kin ... they are counted as cousins. But my husband and I – we are not [kin]. Somehow [we] converge into kin ... But a husband and a wife are not kin – kin are not allowed to marry ... [laugh].' According to her it is better not to marry kin because of genes and it's not recommended for cousins to marry, nor second cousins, not even third cousins. Kristina thinks that a love relationship should not develop if there is a possibility of kin relatedness: 'Of course, looking back – we all have our beginning from Adam and Eve, so we all are kin if we look very, very far back. But the kinship has to be very, very far back in the past.'

In Kristina's narrative on kinship there is a variety of entangled things and matters. People, communication, family, needs, spiritual matters, feelings, ties, kin gatherings, time, kin classification, the real, genes, matrimonial rules, knowledge, Adam and Eve, relationships and relatedness intertwine with each other in her understanding of kinship. In my opinion, it is an eclectic view, but, according to her, 'It is clear to everyone'. This encouraged me to look closer and in doing so I discovered an internal order.

The description of kinship Kristina begins with enumerates people related by filiation, and in this context she mentions 'family'. Later, when she speaks about her brothers and sisters-in-law and explains to me why a husband and a wife are not 'real kin', she speaks about 'kin' and exemplifies kin by cousins – collateral relatives. I suggest that those two different types of relatedness – filial and collateral – are influential categories in local understanding of family (*šeima*) and kinship (*giminystė/giminė*). Based on numerous ethnographic examples, I want to emphasise that, in Lithuanian thinking, the 'family' is understood through filial links and 'kinship' through collateral relatedness where the position of parents and children, on the one hand, and cousins and siblings, on the other, is significant in the ranking of relatives as family or kin members.[5] This structural distinction between 'family' and 'kinship' is also juxtaposed with people's classification of social relationships. Affirming that family and kin relationships are similar in character, our interviewees nevertheless place 'family' within the private and domestic domain, in physical and social proximity as well as everyday interaction, and 'kinship' and 'kin' within the public domain, including festivities and ritual events, kin gatherings and life cycle rituals (Boholm 1983; Holy 1996; Čepaitienė 2003).

Nonetheless, this separation between family and kinship is recognised not in its completeness but in mutual interaction. A middle-aged man, Antanas, in response to the question about a husband and wife says:

> For instance, my brother ... If there is a gathering of the close family circle, say, the family – my sister, brother, my wife, my brother's wife, some of his wife's relatives – we gather together for birthdays. After a drink or so, my brother tells us that 'we kin' have come here together. But then he indicates to his wife and says that she is not actually kin, just as my wife, Silva, is also not my kin. That's how it is. But family is family. And kin are kin. Everything should be kept within bounds ... according to blood relations, a wife should not be kin. But since the children are related to both parents, they bind the two together into kinship.

Mentioning the 'family circle', Antanas enumerates all who, in his view, belong to the family including siblings, spouses and relatives-in-law. But later, after naming this family 'kin', he recalls his brother's words, and regroups people under the criterion of 'blood relations'. This time he separates out spouses – husband and wife – and consequently family and kinship. It looks as if the boundaries were established firmly and with authority. However, after doing that, Antanas once again dismantles the boundary by saying that the appearance of a child creates a kinship bond between a husband and wife and 'bind[s] the two together in kinship (*suriša į giminę*)'.

The discussion finally returns to the same point about the child as a bond uniting a husband and wife. However, this time the binding occurs at a different level – that of kinship. Though husband and wife are not born kin to each other, the child is born kin to both of them and thus links them together and 'create[s] closeness defined in the way familial and kinship relations overlap' (Strathern 1995: 351; see also Schneider 1968). The child transfers the familial relationships into kin relatedness and establishes kin relatedness between a husband and wife, which, however, remains specific – it is not direct, but mediated by the child.

Where Relatedness Is Established Through 'One's Own'

Negotiating the application of ART and the relationship between husband and wife and child, the residents of Kuršėnai often use the idiom of 'one's own': 'one's own child (*savas vaikas*)', 'one's own blood (*savas kraujas*)' or 'one's own genes (*savi genai*)'. They represent the view that sharing of bodily substances in the 'make-up' of a child (Edwards 2005) establishes relatedness, which is based on possession and properties of identity

(Edwards and Strathern 2000; Alber 2003). However, in Lithuanian the word *savas* has a meaning that extends beyond the contents of possession and identity. It refers to 'closeness' (Strathern 1995) and 'subjectivity' (Orobitg and Salazar 2005) and the way in which they are maintained and processed. It means 'belonging to you, grown by you, made by you, being yours and used by you' as well as 'close, not strange' and 'a very close person (kinsman, family member)'.[6]

The idiom of 'one's own' is negotiated in the interviewees' stories about gamete donation and surrogate motherhood. Here the context of ART assists in emphasising both the bodily substances and physical contact necessary in creating the tie (see also Nathalie Manrique, this volume). Sharing the 'mother's genes', being in the mother's body, being affected by certain hormones and being borne by a mother despite sperm or ova donation makes the child the 'mother's own' or 'at least one half is there'. In cases of gamete donation, the women stress that the child nevertheless would contain a portion of the woman who carries and gives birth to it, and they say that, under these circumstances, the child is still 'partly [the mother's] own (*dalis sava*)'. A middle-aged woman, Aldona, says that '[t]he only input in that case is the fact that the child develops in that woman's body. But it would still be affected by certain hormones, it would still bond the child [with her].' This is a powerful argument that rejects surrogate motherhood. Surrogate mothers are seen as new persons who enter into the constitution of a child with their own ways of relatedness. Male interviewees have a similar opinion about a sperm donor. They say that the donation changes the manner of belonging between a father and a child, and transfers the relationship of 'one's own' into 'like one's own (*kaip savo*)'. They see the sperm donor like a 'stranger (*svetimas*)' in the family who through the act of donation 'has sex' with an inseminated woman, brings with him his juridical rights to the child ('the image of parenthood', Hirsch 1993: 78) and his 'genetic tree (*genetinis medis*)' – that is kinship. The only possibility to separate him out is to make him unknown and 'illegal (*nelegalas*)'.

All this, however, brings us to the next question: the child's belonging is established through more than sharing of bodily parts or through physicality. Bodies and substances, in Kuršėnai people's narration, stand not for themselves, but for a person: a man, a woman, a child, a stranger or anybody else identified by name, relations, duties, rights, associations or roots. This is not merely the imagining of the 'personality' of gametes (Martin 1991: 500) but the perception of people indivisible from their physical and social entities (Edwards 2000; 2005). When interviewees speak about sperm, they speak about concrete people with rights of possession, kinship ties, or thoughts and aspirations. When they speak about a child's being in the mother's body or 'carried under the heart (*po širdim nešiotas*)', they speak about particular care and mothering, about the transfer of 'thoughts and something else to the child she is expecting'.[7] To emphasise this, I draw on cases when the bodily experiences are totally ignored by saying that the mother or the parents are not merely those who gave birth, but are those who nurtured and bred a child, who loved and taught it. This intersection of the bodily and the social can be compared with the complexity of the way adopted children are made into kin while taking into account their biological origins, for example, as in Norwegian practices of transnational adoption (Howell 2003; Melhuus and Howell, this volume) or with the way in which physical and moral resemblances are thought to be meaningful in the construction of the body (Marre and Bestard, this volume).

Moreover, this belonging appears to be individual in respect of each of the parents. The child might be the 'mother's own' but not the father's and vice versa. But how then is the child imagined to mediate the relationship and to bind husband and wife together? Interviewees' stories are informative on this. According to Mindaugas there is a kind of sharing of roles in the constitution of the child. The male stands at the beginning – he is 'a provider' of life – and the woman is at the continuation – 'she is only a carrier of life'. Kazimieras, a middle-aged man, tells us more. He says that the child receives intellect from the father, but the majority of inherited traits are passed to the child from the mother who feeds it during gestation through her blood and who has responsibility for the child. He uses the image of 'seed and soil' to describe this, and stresses that 'one receives the harvest from the soil'. In his opinion, if the soil is poor you can plant anything you like, but it will not give you a harvest. The metaphor of 'seed and soil' that he uses is the same as in the accounts from Turkish villagers presented by Delaney (1991: 32–33). When compared, however, it is evident that the meanings differ. Contrary to the stories from the Turkish villages, Kazimieras emphasises not the man's but the woman's role in creating the child, although he says that intellect is passed to the child from its father. Evidently he sees the woman as explicit and active in the child's constitution. I observed the same when speaking with the women. They were more perturbed about the role of the man. As Dalia remarks: '[t]he sperm contains a lot of information. Thoughts and aspirations ... ' Her opinion is in accord with the other woman's thinking when she argues that information about sperm donors should be known and given to the woman undergoing fertility treatment, because she would like to know who the man was who inseminated her.

These cross-images draw on the idea of symmetrical participation in the child's constitution, which is a cornerstone in establishing its relatedness to both parents. The symmetrical projection of a child, although it is oriented to the features of the child, also establishes relatedness between both of them, and the child becomes the mediator of their relatedness. To use a relevant kinship term, it draws on the aspect of bilaterality in defining the child's origin. As one man, Audrius, replied to Darius's question, 'Which side is the stronger?': 'Equal, sure, it is equal. That does not mean that the surname is the father's, so the father's blood relation is stronger. Only a child could love one or another more: the father or the mother, or the grandparents on the father's side.' This quotation presents one more aspect. It shows that the symmetry of cross-images tends to neutralise both the father's and the mother's input into a child, and it creates a child as a new personality which is free to start its relationships anew. The child might justify its belonging to both parents or to one parent, or might stretch relationships further along the lines of kin relatedness recruiting other people, for example, grandparents.

To sum up, I want to emphasise that belonging as 'one's own' is established and managed within a social world where participation in the constitution of a child, as well as the sharing of physicality and of bodily links, is not separable from the whole package of feelings, experiences, events, thoughts and relations: from all the 'materialities', in other words, that compose and process the persons in an entire social and cultural universe with particular histories, physical constitutions, lifestyles, values and beliefs. And the relationship between child and parents, and between husband and wife, is fixed within such a complex of 'materialities'. But is this relationship a fact of kinship? I would say that it is. My interviewees' discussion of gamete donation and surrogate motherhood, occurring under the idiom of 'one's own', is actually a discussion about kinship. Here I would draw on the words of a middle-aged woman, Birut, with whom I spoke about kinship during my first stay in Kuršėnai. In answer to my question 'What is kinship?' she says: 'Kinship is a blood relationship. One's own do not abandon you (*giminystė kraujo ryšys. Savas nepaleidžia*).' These words are about kinship in the idiom of 'one's own' and on its fixing effect.

Concluding Remarks

To conclude, I emphasise that my interviewees' accounts and perceptions of ART are revealed gradually by their moving along thematic links and concerns during the course of our conversations. Their accounts develop from ideas that are overt and on the surface of their everyday thinking, to those which are somewhere deep inside or in unexpected 'places' and which are thought to have nothing to do with the subject under discussion. Conceptions of ART begin from stories about technological innovation and reproduction, but little by little the complexities involved in the making of human relations and persons are included: husband and wife, child, family and the third person. Finally, we reach kinship which was said not to be related to ART at the beginning of our conversation.

Through our discussion with interviewees on ART and kinship, we (as ethnographers) became implicated in the way in which people clarified their connections, belongings and self-identifications. But towards the end of our research we noticed that the stories presented by our interviewees, gave us a view of kinship that looks like a particular type of genealogical schema with different signs that describe types of relatedness and relationships. A husband and a wife, 'who are not kin in the real, actual sense, but somehow become part of the kindred group', are put in the first place and their relationship is marked by a specific equal sign (=). The relationship between ancestors and descendants (children of parents, who in turn reproduce children who are thought to mediate their parents' non-related relatedness) is marked by vertical descending and ascending lines of filiation (|). The lines encircled around the husband and wife constitute a family, which is a close and intimate arrangement. The relationship between siblings, that is brothers and sisters, cousins, uncles and aunts is marked by horizontal lines (–). And this collaterality, extending from ego and repeating over generations, embraces the wide, public and extending domain of kinship.

But, just when this genealogical scheme is on the point of completion, it begins to break down in certain places: the places where people as individual persons are situated. It becomes evident that this view of kinship is not stable because it is two-dimensional, as if projected on to a plane and drawn on paper. Persons, defined through physical, relational and historical entities within the states of both being and making, destroy the two-dimensional picture and instead set a more sophisticated view (Schneider 1968, 1984; Strathern 1992a; Carsten 1995a, 2000a, 2004; Edwards 1999, 2000, 2005; Astuti 2000). As nodal points on the kinship net (Astuti 2000) or loops in a kinship mesh, they share *something essential* which is identified in a person and passed on through persons, and which also constitutes the relation of one to another. It absorbs bodily and social 'materialities', as well as ways of relatedness, through the facts and events of life where relations are extended, cut off, mediated, reproduced or made symbolic. This something essential, which is a part of one in another, establishes a kind of closeness and belonging that people call 'kinship'.

My interviewees and I are able to approach this spatial and multidimensional view of kinship from one 'local' corner. That corner is the place of the 'community' as 'expert' on the issue of ART (Edwards 1999) and it places a child and the relationship between husband and wife in the centre of the story. It implies that the family can be detached from kinship and kinship can make the transition from implicitness to explicitness (Salazar 1999) and from invisibility to visibility.

Notes

I am thankful to my colleague Darius Daukšas – we did the field research together and to all my colleagues in the PUG project for their helpful comments and remarks during the workshops. I also thank Jeanette Edwards, Joan Bestard, Carles Salazar, Marit Melhuus and Anne Cadoret for their valuable comments on earlier drafts of this chapter. I am grateful to Mara Almenas and Geoffrey Vasil-Jakulis for helping with the translation of the interviews and for revising the English version. In particular I am thankful to our interviewees – the residents of Kuršėnai – for their cooperation and hospitality.

1. It is a part of a wider study that investigated public understanding of genetics with respect to ethnicity, family and kinship through research in the community and in clinics, together with the study of legal texts and media

2. items, between 2002 and 2004. This is also supplemented by my previous field experience in a number of small Lithuanian towns and villages during the summers of 1997 and in 1999–2000.
2. I am grateful to Jeanette Edwards for suggesting this idea.
3. In the Lithuanian media and in juridical language ART is called 'artificial insemination (*dirbtinis apvaisinimas*).
4. *Lietuvių kalbos žodynas (Dictionary of Lithuanian Language)*, 1956, Vilnius: Valstybinė politinės ir mokslinės literatūros leidykla, Vol. 3, pp. 309–312; 1986, Vilnius: Mokslas, Vol. 14, pp. 605–8.
5. I would like to thank Anne Cadoret for valuable comments and comparative reflections on the different aspects of family and kinship in French and Lithuanian cases.
6. *Lietuvių kalbos žodynas (Dictionary of Lithuanian Language)*, 1981, Vilnius: Mokslas, Vol. 12, 238–41.
7. The expression 'carried under the heart' is used for the state of being pregnant.

CHAPTER 3

EATING GENES AND RAISING PEOPLE: KINSHIP THINKING AND GENETICALLY MODIFIED FOOD IN THE NORTH OF ENGLAND

Cathrine Degnen

Introduction

With the advent of biotechnology in application to foodstuffs the implications of genetic technologies apply no longer just to human or animal bodies, but also to the food people eat. Likewise, the realm of biotechnology and new genetics with which social scientists have to date been concerned (largely *reproductive* genetic technologies) must now accommodate a new level of intersection: that of genes, body and food. Food is embedded in a complex constellation of social meaning. It has bodily connotations for health and nutrition; it plays a prominent role in identity and belonging; and it has a significant place within macro-level processes of economics, politics and science and technology. What then do questions about genetically modified food permit us to ask and comprehend about public understandings of genetics that research into genetic technologies relating to human reproduction or to therapeutic applications have not yet addressed? What are the implications of public understandings of genetically modified food for notions of relatedness and of kinship?

Kinship Thinking

This chapter is premised on an understanding of kinship as a cultural mode of connectedness that cannot simply be reduced to a form of social organisation, and one in which kinship cannot be 'hived off as a discrete sphere of social life' (Edwards 2000: 27). In particular, I borrow the concept of 'kinship thinking' from Jeanette Edwards (2000) to explore kinship in relationship to food. Kinship thinking is the ways in which connections and relatedness are perceived, selected and employed in everyday life. It includes the culturally and historically variable ways in which people identify connections between them via shared substance (such as blood, gene, flesh or bone), and also includes the making and remaking of 'social relationships through intimacies of care and effort' (Edwards 2000: 27). Edwards further elaborates that kinship thinking is not a static, fixed recipe for forging relations but rather that certain aspects of it are emphasised at certain moments and in certain contexts.

Fruitful questions emerge from pairing kinship thinking with the genetic modification of food: what are the different levels at which genetic modification leads people to think in terms of relatedness and then in terms of dissimilarity? People are always 'eating genes', but when and in what circumstances does this become problematic? What links might kinship thinking reveal between food choices and the intimacies of parental care and effort? My reflections on these questions and the intersecting realms of food, genetic technology and kinship are based on a year of ethnographic fieldwork that I conducted between 2003 and 2004 in the north of England. During this time, I worked with groups of people who, although they did not have expert knowledge on genetic modification, had a great deal of expertise in growing plants and in the production and consumption of food. This research has sought to understand how people make sense of genetically modified food in light of their own situated knowledge and frames of reference.

There are three points of articulation between food, genetic modification and the making of persons and relationships that I will explore here, the first two of which are ethnographic. First, feeding and eating are involved in the reproduction of social relationships, particularly family relationships. Secondly, cultural understandings of the role of food in the making of persons intersect with parental responsibilities in making one's own kind of person. As food and people are points of social intersection and of kinship thinking, genetically modified food may in turn raise relevant and interesting questions about kinship thinking itself.

The third connection to be made between kinship thinking and genetically modified food is an analytical one. This is premised on the argument that with the ascendancy of genetic engineering and genetic technologies, more seems now to be at stake and in question at the boundaries between the biological and the social. Consider for example what Paul Rabinow calls 'biosociality'. In coining this term, Rabinow seeks to draw attention to the implications of the new genetics, operating as it does within a paradigm of modernist rationality that permits a knowing of genetic information in such as way that genes can also be altered and manipulated via biotechnology (Rabinow 1992). While sociobiology used biological metaphors for forging an 'improved' society and thus understood the construction of culture in terms of a metaphor with nature,

Rabinow perceives a ground shift within the emergence of biosociality whereby 'nature will be modeled on culture understood as practice. Nature will be known and remade through technique and will finally become artificial, just as culture becomes natural. Were such a project to be brought to fruition, it would stand as the basis for overcoming the nature/culture split' (Rabinow1992: 241–42). Through techniques that permit the alteration of genes, nature is thus arguably denaturalised. Rabinow posits in turn an emergence of new social identities around things like 'a shared gene', and his oft-cited quote on biosociality above was written with reference to the Human Genome Project, mandated to map and sequence the human genome. My ethnographic work on genetically modified food has prompted me to wonder what biosociality might look like if considered from the perspective of biotechnology when applied to food. What are the possibilities of genetically modified food for 'overcoming the nature/culture split' on the level of everyday practices and understanding?

New genetic technologies also arguably promote paradigms for understanding the world based on 'metaphors of information for understanding the human condition, rather than, as had been the case before, a metaphor of machine. Everything can now be reduced to codes rather than to the nuts and bolts, cogs and wheels' (Green 2002: 192). The rub is, as Green explains, that, unlike mechanical bits and bobs, 'codes look much the same whether they are the genetic code of a human being or the structural code of the videotape containing an episode of The Simpsons' (2002: 192). This sort of framing that melts modernist boundaries between categories previously assumed to be fixed (such as nature/culture, subject/object) has enabled Donna Haraway to argue explicitly that technoscience, the hybridisation of technology and science, is 'a form of life, a practice, a culture, a generative matrix' (1997: 50) in which we are all implicated. This is because technoscience shifts the epistemological, constitutive ground on which we build our understanding of the world. Genetic modification (in all of its various guises) is one manifestation of technoscience that collapses categories which were once perceived as 'true'.

Indeed, Haraway (1997) posits that transgenic entities, by their very presence, change the texture of the world human beings inhabit. Genetically modified food challenges commonly held perceptions of the distinction between nature and culture as separate and separable realms. As an example, Haraway describes an event from May 1994: the granting of approval by the US. Food and Drug Administration for Calgene to market its transgenic Flavr Savr tomato.[1] She writes that transgenic entities like the Flavr Savr 'simultaneously fit into well-established taxonomic and evolutionary discourses and also blast widely understood senses of natural limit' (Haraway 1997: 56). The collapse of these categories means that the distinction between subject (such as a human being) and object (such as a genetically modified tomato) is no longer sustainable. Although these categories may never have been as clear-cut and fixed as Euro-Western thinking agreed to pretend they were,

Haraway argues that divisions and categories will never again even appear to be static (Myerson 2000).

But Haraway has another point to make. This is that, while we are all implicated and knitted into the hybridisation of technology and science because of how it transforms our ways of knowing the world, we are also implicated via kinship. Haraway argues that 'cyborg figures – such as the end-of-the-millennium seed, chip, gene, database, bomb, fetus, race, brain, and ecosystem – are the offspring of implosions of subjects and objects and of the natural and artificial' (Haraway 1997:12). These cyborg figures forge a kinship of entities that include both genetically modified food and human beings, a 'kinship [which] is a technology for producing the material and semiotic effect of natural relationship, of shared kind' (1997: 53). Haraway argues that transgenic entities are new family members: 'By the 1990s, genes are us; and we seem to include some curious new family members at ever [sic] level of the onion of biological, personal, national, and transnational life' (1997: 56). Such 'couplings across taxonomic kingdoms' (1997: 60), which see genes passing from flounders to tomatoes and silk moths to potatoes, are redefining 'the whole system of "kinship relations" within which we live' (Myerson 2000: 17, quoting Haraway 1997: 89). Haraway goes one step further arguing that anything less than a full embrace of these new genetically modified family members would be having recourse to dangerous rhetorics of purity and genetic contamination: terrain that George Myerson calls 'haunted ground' (Myerson 2000: 36) given the despicable histories and contemporary practices of racism, xenophobia and genocide that have been predicated on keeping categories pure (Haraway 1997). This recognition and affirmation of kinship with transgenic entities that Haraway calls for are, on paper, extremely compelling. It also opens up another channel, in addition to the suggestions prompted by the literature on anthropology and (non-genetically modified) food, for thinking through some of the ways in which kinship thinking and genetically modified food may (or may not) go together.

Anthropology, Food and Kinship

Anthropological approaches to food demonstrate how feeding and eating are not neutral practices but are instead laden with cultural and symbolic significance.[2] Food carries symbolic meaning about class, nationality, gender, identity and ethnicity. As with the broader reflexive turn in anthropology to historicise and problematise its object of enquiry, similar theoretical models have been applied to the study of food. Pat Caplan comments how 'foods have histories and ... practices [that] can only be understood in their historical context. Changes in the wider society – such as new ideas [like] ... the relationship between humans and nature ... may be powerfully symbolised by changes in food and eating' (Caplan1997: 8). Sidney Mintz and Christine Du Bois (2002) provide a comprehensive and valuable review of the sub-field of food and eating. After a brief discussion of the history of the study of food in anthropology, which highlights key texts such as Boas's work on Kwakiutl salmon preparation and Lévi-Strauss's structuralist writing on food, Mintz and Du Bois break the literature down into several thematic strands. This includes classic ethnographies on food systems; accounts of single food substances; the impact of social change such as industrialisation and globalisation on food; food insecurity; the connections between food, rituals and belief systems; and the place of food and eating in the construction of identity. Mintz and Du Bois rightly point out that the anthropology of food and eating has been a valuable site for refining theoretical arguments ranging in scope from political economy, cultural materialism and symbolism to the social construction of memory. They attribute the usefulness of food for promoting theoretical advances to the fundamental place that food occupies in human existence and social life.

One topic that is not addressed in their review is the link between kinship and food. Carole Counihan, however, has written about the ways in which 'food is a prism that absorbs and reflects a host of cultural phenomena' (1999: 6) and that studying the meaning people attribute to food, eating and feeding 'enables a holistic and coherent look at how human beings mediate their relationship with nature and each other across cultures and through history' (1999: 7). Counihan elaborates on how 'eating with people is an affirmation of kinship' (Siskind 1973, cited in Counihan 1999: 17), with a connection between food and fostering still held within the etymology of the English language: 'old English "foster" means "food"' (Young 1971, cited in Counihan 1999: 17). Counihan further explains that: 'As humans construct their relationship to nature through their foodways, they simultaneously define themselves and their social world. Through producing, distributing, and consuming food, they act out some of their most important relationships to family, friends, the dead, and the gods. Food provides order to the world and expresses multiple meanings about the nature of reality (1999: 24). Counihan's evocation of the natural and the social and how cultural constructions of them play out through the production, distribution and consumption of food takes on a new level of significance with the emergence of genetically modified food. While food and eating have always been a portal linking the natural and the social, genetically modified food reveals categories that once seemed rigid to be much more unstable, as Haraway, cited above, also demonstrates.

Food and body are intimately linked within Euro-Western thought: when food is ingested into the body, for example, it is perceived as constituting the body. Both 'food' and 'body' already hold, carry and reproduce meaning about society and culture, as well as playing significant roles in the symbolic world that humans use to demarcate social difference and similarity in everyday social life. In Britain, food has also emerged as a political hot potato.[3] Commentators trying to explain the differences between US and UK public responses to genetically modified food have noted that, since the 1980s, Britons have experienced a series of public health scares that have led to a widespread distrust in government agencies' ability and willingness to protect the public.[4] The salmonella scares of the late 1980s, the bovine spongiform encephalopathy (BSE) and variant Creutzfeldt-Jakob disease (CJD) crises of the 1990s and foot-and-mouth disease in 2001 are some of the most obvious examples.

Simultaneously, anthropologists working in Europe have begun noting a recent marked growth of public interest in food politics (Leitch 2003). Alison Leitch, writing about the Slow Food movement in Italy argues that this depth of European concern over food issues and food policy are part and parcel of contested visions of European identity and worries over the changing nature of national boundaries:

> Issues such as the introduction of genetically modified foods and crops ... are now central topics of conversation in most European nations. I would suggest that public anxiety over these risks, both real and imagined, is symptomatic of other widespread fears concerning the rapidity of social and economic change since the Maastricht Treaty of 1992. In sum, food and identity are becoming like the 'Euro', a single common discursive currency through which to debate Europeaness and the implications of economic globalization at the beginning of the twenty-first century (Leitch 2003: 441–42).

Like Mary Douglas's (1970, 1975) work on food and eating, which demonstrates how 'food and eating are symbolic of a particular social order ... [and so] the patterns ... stand for much more than themselves' (Caplan 1997: 2), the issues raised by genetically modified food and the worries over food risks that Leitch identifies above are also connected with turmoil in the social order. Contemporary arguments over genetically modified food are occurring in the midst of other dynamics, such as widespread public mistrust of science and government; willingness of the US government to forcibly promote biotechnology interests in a reluctant Europe via the World Trade Organisation; and communal experiences in the UK of food and health scares. All of these elements are critical contextualising factors to take into consideration when examining public understandings of genetically modified food.

Feeding, Mothering and Responsibility

Returning to the links between food and kinship thinking, ethnographic research offers more clues of the links to be made between parents, children and food cross-culturally. Anne Allison writes about Japanese nursery school children and the boxed lunches, called *obentō*, that their mothers elaborately prepare for them. She traces the ways in which 'mother and child are being watched, judged, and constructed' via both the mother's skill and care in preparing the *obentō* and the child learning to conform to institutional norms of collectivity at the nursery school (Allison 1991: 195). Deviation on the part of either the mother (in preparing the *obentō*) or the child (in eating the *obentō* according to school rules) results in isolating social sanctions and disapproval.

Furthermore, as Allison explains, this is an ideologically loaded practice directed by the state in the nursery schools. Beginning school in Japan is characterised as distressing for children. The *obentō* is perceived as helping to ease this experience for the child and 'allow[s] a child's mother to manufacture something of herself and the home to accompany the child as s/he moves into the potentially threatening outside world' (Allison 1991: 199). Through the assiduous labour of the mother in fashioning her child's lunch box meal, the *obentō* holds symbolic meaning of both mother and home. Maternal responsibility emerges thematically in Allison's account: 'The onus for [the mother] is getting the child to consume what she has made, and the general attitude is that this is far more the mother's responsibility ... than the child's' (1991: 202). If the *obentō* is not prepared properly, the child may fail to eat it (which is a serious offence), or the teacher monitoring the quality of both child and *obentō* will comment upon it, with a quality *obentō* reflecting a quality mother and vice versa. Allison explains how 'it is precisely through this work that the woman expresses, identifies, and constitutes herself' (1991: 203) and also, arguably, helps constitute her child as a fully fledged member of Japanese society.

In another ethnographic site Janet Carsten, writing about Malays on the island of Langkawi, examines notions of feeding, kinship and personhood (1995b). She explains how Malays become both complete persons and also become kin through everyday practices of consuming food together in the residences they share. Carsten argues for an understanding of kinship and personhood which is processual. Focusing on a theme of substance and how it is acquired through feeding, Carsten traces how 'bodily substance is not something with which Malays are simply born and that remains forever unchanged ... [but] it gradually accrues and changes throughout life as persons participate in relationships' (1995b: 225). The substances Carsten has in mind include blood, breast milk and rice. The sharing of these substances between people also signals the presence of a relation.

What is of particular significance for my purposes here is the way in which food and responsibility again emerge as a theme circulating between mothers and children. Carsten explains that incest prohibitions apply to children who have drunk breast milk from the same woman, as to share breast milk from the same woman equates to a sibling relationship between the children (1995b). Local women elaborated on this point in discussions with Carsten:

> the frequency of formal and informal fostering arrangements ... substantially increases the possibility that a child may drink the milk of a woman who is not its birth mother ... It is quite easy to imagine that a child

who has been casually put on the breast of a neighbour or distant kinswoman might later marry her child. This ever-present threat looms large in the minds of the villagers ... If two of the children a woman had breast-fed later married each other, she would bear responsibility for the incest (Carsten 1995b: 227–28).

Mothers' work and actions of feeding are also central to the 'long process of becoming – [of] acquiring substance', as mothers' blood nourishes children in the womb; breast milk is a component of kinship; and the food that women cook in the hearth of the house forges emotional connections that are critically important in order to create relatedness (Carsten 1995b: 234). Carsten concludes that notions of relatedness and kinship amongst Malay in Langkawi are 'not predicated on any clear distinction between "facts of biology" (like birth) and "facts of sociality" (like commensality)', unlike a Schneiderian understanding of kinship which retains an analytical separation between the two categories (1995b: 235). Interestingly, notions of responsibility, food and mothering in the north of England also throw into contention such borders and blur the boundaries between 'facts of biology' and 'facts of sociality'. I turn now to my own ethnographic data to further explore these ideas.

Bodies, Babies and Working Against Contamination

Josie[5] and I were talking about her changing relationship with food over her lifetime. She lives in Wilmslow, Cheshire, to the south of Manchester, and works in the tourism and heritage industry. In her early forties, Josie is also married with children, and over the course of her life has lived in several parts of Britain as well as abroad. Josie tells me that when she went away to university, she did not know anything about cooking and how it was a bit of a shock to realise that preparing meals involved work and skill that were taken-for-granted aspects of living in the parental home and not easily replicated outside it:

> I do remember the feeling of 'oh gosh, I have been used to having really, really, nice, good food' and this idea of when you are young, you take it for granted, and it doesn't hit you until you've had another miserable day with, you know, Bean Feast,[6] and sort of appreciating going back for weekends and holidays and having really nice food on tap, as it was!

She then makes an immediate and striking transition in her narrative account from thinking about her own perception of food as a first-year university student (compared with when she still lived at home) to another significant shift in her thinking about food upon the birth of her first child:

> And certainly when Anna was born, I [had been vegetarian at that point for eight years] so when she was born and when she started wanting to eat solids, I really did think 'what do I want to give her?' because I sort of felt

Eating Genes and Raising People 53

> that, well, it's a dilemma. Do you choose what you [have been eating to give to them] or do you make the decision for them about whether they eat meat or not? But I certainly did think, you know, you've got this tiny little baby with perfect skin and bright eyes and you think, you know, do you want to give it crap? And you really don't. It's like sort of defouling [sic] something, you know, you feel really, it's really evident that what you put into her – I think it used to strike me as a bit revolting when you'd see another young baby eating or chewing something that you thought was, [shudders] ... you know, it was absolutely typical, you'd go around in town or something and you'd see little kids being given ... really sort of greasy bakery sausage roll things and they'd be chewing on that and I'd think 'you don't know what is in that!' ... It always used to look, it used to have something, ugh, well, something repulsive about it. So it did, it really did make me think [about] what we gave to Anna.

Josie makes several overlapping and highly relevant points here. The first reaffirms common-sense Euro-Western ideas of 'you are what you eat', with bodies being constituted by what is put into them. A second theme that emerges, however, is the less often articulated but equally critical point of who is doing the feeding and how particular kinds of relationships are forged between parents and children through food. For example, in the case of Josie's university years, she came to recognise a symbolic and emotional difference between 'miserable days' and 'Bean Feast' while alone at university, compared with 'really, really, nice, good food', 'on tap', prepared and eaten in the familial home. Thirdly, a clear theme arises of parental responsibility for protecting the purity of children's bodies through monitoring food choices: in Josie's language, of 'perfect skin' and 'bright eyes' versus 'defouling' [sic] with 'repulsive' 'greasy bakery sausage roll things'. Food is a conduit of transmission, as Josie explains. When between parent and child, food is in particular a conduit for building the kind of baby one wants with responsibility on the shoulder of the parents for making the 'right' kinds of food choices.

Indeed, in general terms, parents (and particularly mothers) spoke about their children and food choices in very elaborated ways. A second example comes from a woman I have named Julia. She lives in Barnsley, South Yorkshire, and is a single mother in her late thirties who after many years of part-time jobs and full-time mothering is now studying for a university degree. We started by talking about how food has changed since she was growing up and the extremely tight budget she remembers her mother having to try and feed the family on. Talk then turned to Julia's own experiences as a mother and her concerns when her son, at the age of two, began to refuse food. After two years of trying to persuade a very finicky eater to eat more she brought him, in desperation, to the doctors:

Julia   When he were four, because it went on for years, this, I took him to the doctors, I said 'Look, he's so thin and all he'll eat is custard creams!'[7]
Cathrine   He wouldn't eat like, bananas or, I don't know, toast?

Julia	He'd eat, if I had something on my plate, he'd eat something off my plate, tentatively. He used to like finny haddock.
Cathrine	What's that?
Julia	It's smoked haddock; I used to fold it in a piece of bread and put it in his mouth and he loved that but he wouldn't have any for himself. Just very strange eating habits, really decisive about what he didn't like. And the doctor said, 'When he's hungry, he'll eat, don't worry about it. He's obviously developing properly, getting nourishment from somewhere.' I persisted trying to introduce other kinds of food ... if you made a meal and put it on the table he just wouldn't eat any of it ... but it were such a worry for me because I wanted him to eat. I wanted him to grow and develop and feed his brain and things and I were like 'he's not eating, he's only eating custard creams!' He used to revert back to these custard creams, it went on for years and years. It was just like a mealtime anxiety thing for me, but I tried not to transfer it over to him, I used to say 'just taste this' ... but the lips would go [pursing her own lips as an example] and that would be it! There would be nothing going in there.

Julia, faced with a finicky eater, felt she had far less autonomy with her child's food choices than did Josie. Despite this, the sense of responsibility and urgency over her son's eating weighed heavily and more than ten years later still animated her greatly.

This will at first glance seem a banal point to raise as of course a parent is both responsible and, ideally, interested in what her or his child is consuming. 'We are what we eat' and the threat of malnutrition or poor health in one's child from lack of food and nutrition seems to be a fairly straightforward equation. I believe, however, that while these cultural ideals are playing out, there are other notions simultaneously at work.

I propose that perception of parental responsibility is also informed by ideas of what kind of person they are responsible for shaping, and that the sort of food their children are ingesting reflects on both the character and respectability of the parent but also the larger project of making kin and making children. Josie does not like the 'greasy sausage rolls' she sees children being fed on the streets during a morning's shopping in town; Julia wishes her son would eat food that would help 'develop and feed his brain' rather than his proclivity for highly processed custard cream biscuits, something she does not consider to merge with her idea of what is good for growing a healthy, smart son.

While the narrative examples above from Josie and Julia are excerpts from longer interviews about food and understandings of genetically modified food, neither of these two interviewees explicitly addressed children, parenting and genetically modified food. This next narrative passage from a third mother does however make such links explicit:

Cathrine	Do you think that organic food can be genetically modified?

Pamela	No.
Cathrine	It's just not possible for the two to be held together?
Pamela	No. Organic food to me means as nature designed it. As our bodies have been designed to accept it. You know, it's not anything that *we* can mess around with, it's ... you know, I believe that the foods that our bodies cope the best with are things that have always been here and you're less likely to have any problems as a result of that. So I can't accept it.
Cathrine	And is organic food, I mean do you remember how your relationship with it developed? Is it something that evolved gradually over time?
Pamela	I think having a child makes the difference to people. To us it certainly made us think 'you have something that is not contaminated by anything' and you don't want to sully that at all. That certainly is an issue. We get a lot of young mothers [in the shop] looking for organic food for their children; they don't necessarily eat it themselves, but they want their babies to have it. That's why, I mean, organic baby food is huge.

Pamela is a mother of two in her late thirties and works full-time. She and her husband own and run an organic health food store to the south of Manchester. Although this means that they are both more actively (and also professionally) engaged with issues surrounding food production, genetic modification technology and organic food than most people who partook in this research, the points Pamela raises are not unrepresentative of views expressed during my fieldwork. Ever-increasing sales of organic food in Britain, but particularly of organic baby food, attest to this. Indeed, a national UK newspaper, the *Guardian* (5 November 2003), recently reported that three out of every four British babies are now eating organic food (although whether or not this was processed food or fresh is not clear) on a regular basis, reflecting Pamela's experiences at her health food shop.

Mothers like Josie, Julie and Pamela express concerns over what their children are eating. This is perhaps in part due to Euro-Western explanatory models that agree 'we are what we eat' and consequently that children's diets must be balanced and nutritious in order to promote health and growth. The point I wish to make here is that food choice in this context is less about choosing healthy foods or risk analysis calculations[8] and more about how exercising food choices for one's child imbricates parents in kinship thinking via food. My attention is arrested by the ways in which parents participating in this research elaborated on the essence of their offspring in relation to the food choices they had to make for them, and what this in turn 'brings into focus', to borrow a phrase from Edwards (2000: 104). The first characteristic brought into focus is how one's own children are perceived as pure, uncontaminated and unexposed to detrimental and polluting agents. Maintaining this state of purity in one's children through careful consideration of what they are eating, and sometimes by critical reflection on the implications of genetic technologies and food, emerges as a priority for British parents.

The second characteristic relates to two critical kinship questions Edwards raises in the Introduction to this volume: 'what constitute[s] relatedness between kin' and what are understandings of how people are 'created and grown'. Authors such as Counihan have demonstrated that feeding and eating forge and reproduce social relationships amongst family members and wider social connections. The examples I have used from the north of England, Japan and Langkawi confirm this, but they also bring into focus another detail: how relatedness between parents and children is also partly constituted by feelings of responsibility for monitoring what one's children are eating. I do not wish to go so far as to make claims for universality based on this evidence, but the recurrence of the theme is a striking link between three culturally distinct field sites.

What I shall argue is that, at least in the north of England, relatedness between parents and children is partly forged through notions of responsibility via making food choices on behalf of one's children. Food is perceived as constitutive of both body and person and some food is perceived as befouling/defiling the inherent 'purity' of children's bodies. This is a threat to work against as part of the project of being and becoming a parent. Such material calls to mind Carsten's argument about the blurred boundaries between 'facts of biology' and 'facts of sociality': feeding and eating make people belong via both realms in the north of England[9] as much as they do in Langkawi. Parents like Pamela describe themselves as striving not to 'sully' the bodily purity of their children, and parental responsibility for making the right choices for dependent children is a heavy one. Making the right food choices figures as one element in a myriad of decisions in how best to 'grow' one's children. Making food choices is also to engage in a process of making people and, specifically, making one's own people, which continues after conception and birth. What people eat and who they eat it with have rightly been identified as elements of creating family, but this material highlights how relatedness between kin, particularly between parent and child, is also constituted via the tropes of responsibility for and monitoring of food choices. This is kinship thinking in the shopping trolley, in the kitchen and on the dinner plate.

I have up to now been arguing that kinship and relatedness are built via notions of parental responsibility for the quality of children's food consumption (though, of course, what counts as a valued food varies) as both desirable and undesirable characteristics can be transmitted through the conduit of food. Genetically modified food, as Pamela explains, is one category that by and large is not seen as conducive to this project.[10] This is a thread linking food choices, kinship thinking and genetically modified food at an individual level. I would like now to take a further step in examining more communal levels of experience and how, via food choices, kinship, in a rhetorical sense, is denied to genetically modified food while simultaneously forging a relatedness at the level of community and 'the public'.

Genetic Modification, Connectedness and Communal Experience

When I began my ethnographic fieldwork on public understandings of genetically modified food, I anticipated that the people involved in the project would have a great deal to say about the topic of genetically modified food. The issue was receiving heavy media attention in 2003 with field test crop trials sponsored by the government coming to an end (and still being ripped up from the fields in which they were growing by protesters). The government was also busily launching a three-stranded review of the technology including a widely advertised public consultation exercise in the summer of 2003 called 'GM Nation?'.[11] The *Daily Mail*, a popular and Conservative tabloid newspaper, had launched a campaign against genetically modified foods and two broadsheets, the *Guardian* and the *Independent*, were running regular coverage of stories on genetic modification.[12] Britain appeared to be a nation gripped by worries over genetic modification. If the newspapers were any indication to go by, it seemed as though food, being something everyone eats and feeds their children, and the implications of genetically modifying it, were topics that everyone would have a strong opinion on.

I discovered instead a much more complicated terrain (Degnen 2006). Many people with whom I spoke were often reluctant to engage in discussions on the topic, saying that it was something they knew nothing about. This example comes from the beginning of an interview I conducted with a woman in her sixties living in the Barnsley area whom I had known for almost five years at the time of the interview: 'But, see, we don't know! We don't know anything about it at all, full stop, *nothing*. I couldn't tell you now what GM foods are. I couldn't tell you. Haven't a clue.' Indeed, many of the interviews and informal conversations I conducted with a wide range of people (in terms of age, area of residence, socio-economic background and gender) began with my interlocutor professing no knowledge of genetic modification, surprise at my wish to speak to them about the topic and an urge to clarify that they were not well-informed on the topic. Some people who participated in the research were more comfortable discussing the topic, and although they were a small minority, many of these people were better informed than I was on the ins and outs of information on, figures about and politics over genetic modification. Furthermore, although the majority of people involved in this project were sceptical about the application of genetic technology to food, it is important to point out that this was not universally true and some participants felt highly favourable towards genetic modification as both desirable and necessary.

Although genetic modification has attracted growing attention in the social sciences (Grove-White et al 1997, 2000; ESRC 1999; Murcott 1999; Shaw 1999, 2002; Heller 2002; Levidow 2002), there is a significant lack of work that situates ideas about genetically modified food ethnographically within the social nature of food and eating. Instead, in the literature, genetically modified food has largely been abstracted from the cultural environments within which it is 'consumed'. Furthermore, most research on understandings of genetically modified food has also mainly focused on 'experts' of various kinds in areas such as food production and retailing, activism, microbiology, biotechnology and government regulation (e.g. Murcott 1999; Shaw 1999; Heller 2002; Lezaun 2004). While researching understandings of genetically modified food with power brokers is instructive, one of the key objectives of the research upon which this chapter draws was to explore the under-investigated everyday sites of discourse and practice.

Of particular relevance to my purposes here are the conceptual linkages people make when discussing genetically modified food. One example out of many is this passage from an interview I conducted in the Barnsley area with a family of three. Ray and Pat, both in their sixties and working for the council, their daughter, Kay, a schoolteacher in her thirties, and I were in the midst of a long conversation about genetically modified food and food changes more generally throughout their lifetimes. We had been talking about whether or not they trusted the government to act in their best interests (the consensus was 'no') when Pat said:

Pat	I don't know, really, I don't really understand why they are wanting to push it. Especially when it's so unpopular.
Cathrine	Tony Blair keeps saying that if we don't keep at the forefront of this new technology then we're going to fall behind and we're not going to be experts in it and …
Pat	Well, tough! I mean …
Ray	But we'll still be living in another two hundred years. These that's going over to GM crops, they might end up dying out!
Kay	Well, it's like with the thalidomide, everybody thought it was the wonder drug, didn't they, until the babies started being born and I don't know, are they going to say in sort of fifty years' time, oh why on earth did we do that, why did we build those schools with asbestos stuffed in them, you know, what a daft idea that was … I think it's a similar thing, isn't it. Is the government really *sure* that it is safe?

Kay here compares genetically modified food and crops to prescribing thalidomide to pregnant mothers before the effects of the drug on the growth of newborn children were understood. She also compares it to the use of asbestos in public buildings such as schools, where children were unknowingly exposed to its carcinogenic properties.

In a different interview, this time with a woman named Lindsay in her twenties living in Cheshire and working in a historical museum, other negative experiences of collective problems were evoked. I asked her what genetic modification makes her think of and she responded:

Lindsay   It makes me very sceptical. It makes me very sceptical of interfering with food in any way, shape or form. I mean, you only have to look at the programme I was watching the other night about mother's milk and the pesticides and the things that are coming out now to affect a younger generation and it's a question of 'Do you know what you're doing with GM food that might occur you know, fifty years down the line, have you actually looked into how its going to affect the nation in every way, shape and form fifty years down the line?' I don't think enough's been done to sort of check that out before they put it on public sale. It's sort of like 'Oh, we found this marvellous thing that means we can improve the amount of food and the quantity of food but we haven't checked about any side effects or occurrences that might happen in twenty-five, thirty years.' You know, the next generation, they're just sort of going to throw it at you.

Narratives about genetically modified food often start with self-deprecating statements of a lack of knowledge about genetic technology in general and genetic modification of food in particular. Despite this, as these narratives unfold, people remember and draw upon shared, communal knowledge forged through experiences of science and technology gone awry to situate their understandings of genetically modified food and the modified genes that they might be ingesting. Thalidomide, asbestos and pesticides in breast milk are held in common by being examples of national and global misadventures with technology or medical science. People evoked these and many other examples in order to explain their disquiet and suspicion about genetically modified food, including DDT, growing resistance to antibiotics, carcinogenic food additives, BSE, myxomatosis, X-rays and cigarettes.

One of the frames of reference within which many people place genetically modified food, then, is a range of examples from past experience where haste in introducing new products and techniques had negative, unforeseen consequences. Additionally, these are historical events that were not usually experienced as a personal health crisis or individual trajectory. Rather, all had ramifications that were borne communally. Genetically modified food, then, is categorised as another example of scientific endeavour potentially outstripping its ability to handle unforeseeable consequences. I argue that this is a communal body of knowledge forged through experience and drawn on in times of uncertainty to evaluate products and practices with socially shared implications. Instead of reaching out towards genetically modified foods and crops as a kinship of beings with much in common with contemporary human experience, people by and large expressed a cautious urge instead to pull up the drawbridge, and apply the test of time to genetically modified food and crops.

Returning to Haraway's arguments explored earlier in this chapter, her cautions against racist thinking strike me as useful in that they keep us on our toes. They keep us thinking critically and thinking in webs of meaning rather than in simple binary modes. But they are also challenging and difficult. Does she really mean that discrimination is universally equal and that human-on-human genocide and holocausts compare equally to a distaste for mixing genetic material in the laboratory, soil and air? Does her argument unintentionally end up belittling the lived consequences of terror inflicted on one group by another? Or is this too simplistic a reaction to the more complicated threads of her argument about notions of purity and impurity (see also Campbell, this volume) and notions of maintaining categories?

As genetic technologies are not abstract ideas but concrete practices producing concrete entities, Haraway's points are highly relevant. However, reading her account chafes slightly because of the disjuncture between her argument and my ethnographic experiences in the north of England. The categories of purity that are being ruptured by technoscience more generally and by genetic modification in particular are not human versus human but human versus non-human; Haraway would argue that such distinctions are now irrelevant given that everything is code, but people on the ground in Barnsley and Wilmslow do not agree. They perceive 'scientists' as choosing to push limits (and all categories have limits or boundaries) for the pleasure of it, for the thrill of it and without regard to the consequences, which have implications for the general public and for the general public's children.

Furthermore, contrary to Haraway's proposition of a new kinship with genetically modified beings, the people I consulted seem to want to keep the boundaries sharp between nature and culture in terms of food. A recurring theme in public understandings of genetically modified food is that people insist on the boundaries between what is 'natural' and what is 'unnatural'. That is to say, while searching for words to describe the process of genetic modification, people often referred to it as 'messing around with nature', 'interfering with nature' or as 'forcing' plants to do something that they are not 'supposed to do'. Language like 'interfering' and 'messing' with nature reveals cultural ideas about how some things, such as genes, may belong in a realm that 'should' be kept separate from human intervention. Mixing genes from different biological kingdoms, such as animals and plants, was particularly categorised as unnatural and undesirable. Fears were raised about the unpredictability of changes to genetic structures once they were no longer within the confines of the laboratory and could instead potentially mix in unintended ways with air, soil, other plants and bacteria. Genetic modification was broadly perceived as altering the 'natural' order of things and the technologies being developed on plants are of the same order as what could in the future be used on people, which was seen as distasteful and a step too far. With regard to biosociality, then, these desires of people participating in this research to keep things 'pure' point not so much to an 'overcoming' of the nature/culture split that Rabinow evokes but rather to a reaffirmation and entrenchment of maintaining these boundaries and categories.

Conclusions

Sarah Franklin proposes that the new genetics is about 'assembling parts that belong to different orders of phenomena according to a logic of totality that is not to be found in the parts, but in the principles, forces and relations that connect the parts' (2003: 82). The question of what is brought together and what is held apart in terms of social and biological connections is at stake in the new genetics. Kinship thinking and thinking about kinship are two ways into these sticky questions. I argue here that genetically modified food demonstrates how such wranglings are not restricted to realms that are explicitly about making families, but are also about making people, making one's own people, making collective decisions about technoscience and making decisions about the boundaries between potential kin. Edwards has explored how kinship and kinship thinking are made out of a complex interplay of being both born and bred (2000). One element of kinship thinking that I have explored here is food choice and parental (particularly maternal) responsibility. Many other elements are simultaneously at work in people's understandings of relatedness and how it is made, but I have chosen to focus on the under-explored dimension of food. Food choices and parental responsibility are both part of a person's upbringing. Both also play a part in reproducing persons, persons who are born pure and in whom much time and consideration are invested in not 'sullying'.

A second perspective on kinship thinking developed here is the thinking about connections and disconnections provoked by GM and food but not in the way Haraway predicts. In my ethnographic experiences, what people want to keep connected and what they want to keep separate are different from what Haraway foresees. 'Couplings across taxonomic kingdoms' (Haraway 1997: 60) are a collapse of boundaries that particularly worried people consulted in the north of England when discussing genetically modified food. To better explain themselves as to why GM food and transgressing species boundaries provoked unease, people made couplings of their own in order to frame their unease with genetic modification. They brought together multiple examples of products, drugs and techniques that had gone awry and incurred collective negative consequences. In so doing, I argue that one more form of kinship thinking is being mobilised: far from being 'ignorant' and 'uneducated' about technoscience, public understandings of genetically modified food that contextualise these new products within a nexus of previous misadventures demonstrate just how thinking and reflective the general public is about GM food. Sophisticated models are being employed which are able to question the intentionality and purpose of technoscience, models that also perceive just how born and bred genetic technologies themselves actually are.

Notes

My research for this chapter and the intellectual environment fostering it were funded under EU Framework 5 and the Quality of Life and Management of Living Resources Programme (contract number QLG 7-CT-2001-01668), 'The Public Understanding of Genetics: a Cross-Cultural and Ethnographic Study of the "New Genetics" and Social Identity' whilst I was a post-doctoral research associate in Social Anthropology at the University of Manchester. I would like to thank the PUG team for vibrant and stimulating conversations which have lasted over two years and are still continuing. Thanks in particular are due to Ben Campbell, Jeanette Edwards, Marit Melhuus, Carles Salazar, Pat Spallone and Katharine Tyler for their questions and comments as this chapter took shape in various incarnations. Last, but by no means least, I would like to acknowledge and thank all of the people who took part in the fieldwork that this chapter represents, giving so generously of their time, energy and patience.

1. The Flavr Savr tomato was genetically altered to delay ripening and was the first commercialisation of a genetically modified organism.
2. A substantial body of literature on the anthropology of food exists. As an introduction to this body of work, see Messer (1984) and Mintz and Du Bois (2002) for comprehensive reviews of the literature, both published in the *Annual Review of Anthropology*.
3. Some would argue 're-emerged', as much historical work has been done on the political place of food such as food riots in Britain. As a starting point, see E.P. Thompson (1993).
4. See, for example, Reilly and Miller (1997).
5. All people referred to here have been assigned pseudonyms and other steps have been taken to preserve their anonymity. The fieldwork was multi-sited and conducted in two areas in the north of England, chosen for the breadth of socio-economic and historical profiles that each represents. The first site, Barnsley, is an area that was heavily industrialised for nearly two centuries due to coal mining, but the closure of the coal mines in the late 1980s and early 1990s has transformed Barnsley beyond recognition on both experiential and socio-economic levels. The second site, the Wilmslow area, is located in the county of Cheshire, one of the wealthiest areas of the UK, with all indices of socio-economic comfort well above national averages, including in education, occupation, income and house prices. The area today is broadly the domain of wealthy 'nouveaux-riches' and middle-class 'professional' families. Despite significant differences in education, employment and income profiles, both areas are, however, remarkably similar ethnically, with over 98 per cent of the population in both boroughs identifying as white. Seeking meaningful social circumstances within which to discuss GM food, I worked with people across a wide spectrum of age, gender, social class and occupation, including gardeners, students, allotment holders, caterers, housewives, health food store owners, farmers, activists and a wide range of professionals not involved in food or science. Some of these people had no vested interest in genetic modification, and others (such as the

activists, farmers and health food store owners) were deeply involved in the debates over GM food.
6. Previous to our interview, on another occasion Josie had described Bean Feast to me as a fairly basic bean and rice casserole from a packet that she learned to make from a flatmate. The dish seems to be low on taste and appeal but high on convenience.
7. A type of biscuit.
8. Although see Caplan (1997: 17–24) for a useful overview of critical perspectives on food, healthy eating, choice and risk.
9. See also Edwards (2000).
10. Although what 'GM' stands for in comparison with 'organic' food is not always so clear-cut. For an exploration of this, see Degnen (n.d.).
11. The other two strands were a scientific review and an economic review.
12. For example, in the six months between 1 May 2003 and 1 November 2003, the *Guardian* and the *Observer* ran 109 items (including articles, opinion pieces, editorials and letter pages) on the topic of GM. Not included in this figure are the dozen or so additional political cartoons that also appeared.

CHAPTER 4

THE FAMILY BODY: PERSONS, BODIES AND RESEMBLANCE

Diana Marre and Joan Bestard

Introduction

The aim of this chapter is to analyse the meanings of resemblance within the context of the Catalan family. Resemblance expresses continuity between individuals and is a good starting point for reflecting on how the constitution of a person through kinship is not limited to isolated individuals, but refers to people that relate to one another. It is our hypothesis that family resemblances are not a true confirmation of the biological truths of kinship but rather are linked to the relational aspect of kinship and to a way of constructing bonds between people. We analyse resemblance as a way of creating continuities between individual persons in a kinship network and also as a way to visualise the double face of Euro-American kinship in the body: that is, what is given and what is made in the constitution of the individual person.

We analyse the significance of family resemblance in the construction of kinship links within Catalan adoptive families. Family resemblance shows continuity among individuals and constitutes a good opportunity for reflecting on the construction of a person through kinship and for making explicit the way in which there is always something given, something non-intentional, in the definition of a person as a relative. Modell points out, in the context of resemblance between parent and adopted in North America, that:

> [they] give the impression of an absolute bond, and an impression counts for a lot in substantiating fictive kinship. In recent decades, the resemblance of an adopted child to her adopting parents gives the impression that her 'genetic make-up' is close to that of her adoptive family – and such

closeness, too, is considered all to the good ... From the point of view of professionals who arrange and finalize adoptions, the family that looks like all others promises to be secure and enduring. (Modell 2002: 6)

The interest in how a child resembles other family members is part of the culture of Catalan family life. It is a way of placing children in a family network and of establishing ties between members of the family. This family resemblance, however, does not necessarily refer exclusively to genetic inheritance. It is not enough to find family resemblance through genetic connection. Rather it is a way of constructing relations in a network of already existing relatives, a way of placing the new body into the group of the family body and constructing the new individual body as a family member. Hence, from an ethnographic point of view, physical resemblance is related to conceptions of embryo formation, to ways of naming and to the transmission of moral character (Vernier 1999). 'Resemblance, in other words, is a socially constructed lens through which "family members" are viewed' (Modell 2002: 22, n. 11).

When Catalan families talk about inheritance they refer to specific physical characteristics (the colour of the eyes, the shape of the nose, the texture of the hair and so on) and constitution (weight and longevity, amongst other things), as well as behaviour patterns (temperament, character, personality). When they look at a newborn baby, they say that she 'takes after' such a person in the family in one aspect and 'takes after' another in another aspect, showing thus a 'consubstantiation' with the family body. According to their view resemblance is not an issue that refers exclusively to genetic transmission. Acknowledging shared physical identities, people maintain moral ties and intimate relations between family members.

The resemblance of a child to different members of the family is an important element in the formation of individual identity. It has to do with processes of identification. According to Freud, in one of his earlier papers, identification is a relational aspect of the person. 'The identification is known in psychoanalysis as the earliest manifestation of an affective tie with another person ... the earliest and most primitive form of the affective tie ... the identification attempts to form the ego analogously to the person used as model' (Freud 2003 [1920]: 43–45). Nevertheless, this resemblance is not exclusively biological; it can be, at the same time, physical and/or moral. 'In these identifications the ego sometimes copies the beloved person and sometimes, on the contrary, the non beloved one ... identification is but partial and highly limited, contenting itself [sometimes] with taking only one feature from the object-person' (Freud [1920] 2003: 43–45).

This chapter is based on anthropological fieldwork carried out primarily in Catalonia, Spain, where we conducted in-depth interviews with married and unmarried couples, single parents and gay and lesbian couples about processes of assisted conception and international adoption. Following Melhuus and Howell (this volume), we also consider that both these ways of obtaining a child belong to the domain of assisted procreation. The interviews were complemented by participant observation in various social networks, principally in associations that focus on issues of assisted procreation and have been established since the second half of the 1990s. As part of our fieldwork, we also conducted participant observation in the Internet lists and chat rooms of these associations, which attract a wider Spanish population.

Kinship and Family Resemblance

Kinship studies have shown how, in Euro-American kinship, nature and culture meet in different ways in the constitution of the intimate relations of the family. Perceived physical resemblances between family members are an ethnographic window through which to analyse the different ways in which nature and culture are mobilised when people refer to their relatives. The fact that physical resemblances between people are cultural perceptions of identity recognition was shown clearly by Malinowski (1932) for the Trobriand Islanders. Malinowski emphasised the differences between his received knowledge of perceiving resemblances between kin and how Trobrianders perceived resemblance. In spite of his own idea that resemblance is related to blood shared between relatives after conception, Trobriand children do not resemble their matrilineal relatives. A person looks like his or her father because it is the child's father who moulds him or her during pregnancy, despite the fact that, according to Trobriand understandings, the father does not share physiological substance with his offspring. Furthermore, it is offensive to say that somebody resembles their mother or their mother's relatives – a maternal uncle, for example – because it is the father who moulds the fetus. To suggest a physical resemblance between an infant and its mother would be to imply that an incestuous relationship had occurred. This connection cannot be made, since in Trobriand society the physical resemblance reveals the non-matrilineal aspect of reproduction, which, contrary to Western ideas about the formation of the body, has nothing to do with conception.

In Western traditions, family resemblances have their origins in conception and they raise the paradoxical question of belonging to a family body and being, at the same time, an individual person. As a whole person he or she is an individual, but as a member of a family this individual receives different inherited traits from different family members. Family genealogies can be perceived in the different physical and moral traits of a newborn, but how they mould newborns in their relationships with others constitutes them as individual persons. As individual agents, they mould themselves through their life cycle. While they receive traits from different members of their family and they identify themselves with some family characters, they are also whole persons and individuals who are different from other family members. In this sense, as Telfer points out, 'practices in and around adoption render visible various cultural processes, notions and forces concerning kinship, identity and relatedness' (Telfer 1999: 145), just as in other fields in new kinship studies.

Many adoptive families' narratives are concerned with various forms of 'kinship links building'. They find some elements of resemblance with the adopted child and through them they begin the process of relating to the child. 'Resemblances essentialize the tie, make it inherent, inevitable, and enduring' (Modell 2002: 8).

Adoptive parents look for and find some previous connection in order to create an enduring relation – a sense of destiny. A mother waiting to collect her daughter in Haiti said that she thought she would have some news on 20 February. She spent that day checking her email every fifteen minutes, but none arrived. However, she had a big surprise when later she learned that the girl assigned to her was born on the 20th of February. Another woman, whose child came from Morocco, said that the child she was given was born on the day she submitted her application. The mother of a child found on a railway line in Kinshasa said that this meant that the girl was going to travel (Howell and Marre 2006). In these narratives adoptive parents reveal one of the main assumptions of kinship, namely that relatedness is something previously given and needs to be activated in order to create a concrete relationship between individuals. Kinship is always a previous relation: it comes from the past, and it is important to discover preceding connections in order to construct future relations with a child. When the new body lacks these prior connections through conception, some other previous relations have to be found on which to build the enduring and intimate solidarity of kinship.

Do Family Resemblances Confirm Kinship?

We begin by presenting, in detail, the case of Asha, the protagonist in one of the first international adoptions in Catalonia. She is a woman in her mid-thirties, adopted when she was seven from an Indian orphanage. Her adoptive family had adopted another Indian girl a few years before her and this girl had never looked for her biological family. By contrast, Asha has written two books retelling in detail her journey and her experience of searching for her biological family including her reunion with them. Asha's first book, published in 2003, was a best-seller and it remained on the top list for many months. At that time, she explained that her book was the result of her interest in telling her story or, as she put it, the 'need to explain myself and to put my experience at the disposal of those persons who may find it useful' (Miró 2003: 123). The book was presented at different public meetings, many of them organised by associations of adoptive families. In her first book, written seven years after her first visit to India, she retells her experience as an adopted daughter and her coming back to India to look for a story about her origins mainly from the nuns of the orphanage where she had lived. The book is dedicated 'To my parents, Josep Miró and Electa Vega', a reference to her adoptive parents, and 'To Radhu and Shevhai, who gave me life', a reference to her biological parents (or, as we would come to know later, those who were believed to be her biological parents). These references were commented upon and criticised by many adoptive parents.

Because of the enormous and rapid success of her two books (Miró 2003, 2004), Asha became a public figure frequently invited on television shows and to social gatherings and not only those related to international adoption. She carried out these presentations and invitations so successfully that she became one of the faces of the *Forum of Cultures 2004* in Barcelona and a famous Catalan TV presenter. She highlighted her preferences for certain clothes and habits linked to an 'Indian' style. Asked, for example, about her preferences for brightly coloured clothes and frankincense, she explained and justified it by her 'genetic inheritance': 'Going to my country of origin and getting to know my origins meant understanding certain attitudes coming from the genetic background that I have. It was very revealing' (Martínez 2004).

Asha's second book was the product of her second visit in search of her biological family when she went along with a team of cameramen and her editorial agent. This time she found a sister whose name, she was surprised to find out, was also Asha. She was told that when she was left in the orphanage her biological father had changed the name given her at birth, which was Usha, to Asha, her sister's name, in the hope of a better future. It was because of this that she entitled her second book *The Two Faces of the Moon*. This is what Asha Miró says about family resemblance in her second book: 'My little nephews, Bausaheb and Rahul, are very much like me. We look so much alike that somebody mentioned that they could easily be taken for my sons. They resemble me physically, even more than their mother, but we are also alike in the way of looking and of talking and when making some gestures' (Miró 2004: 65). Through physical resemblances and gestures she recognises a sense of belonging to the same family. But she goes further, finding physical resemblance between herself and people living in the same places as her biological family. 'I recognise myself, at all times, in the faces of the people from Kolpewadi and Shasha. I know that some of them have my same blood and a similar genetic pattern. They also recognise me as a member of their family' (Miró 2004: 73–74).

Asha was surprised by this because she had always believed that, for sure, she would not have 'anything in common' with her biological family because her 'gestures are Mediterranean'. She had thought that being brought up in Barcelona had kept her 'totally apart from those with whom I share a mother, a father, grandparents, common ancestors'. It is interesting to note that, despite the fact that in many others parts of her books she habitually speaks of 'parents' or 'adoptive parents' and of 'biological parents' as those who 'gave her the life', in this case, she refers to these latter parents without the word 'biological'. It is at this time that she explicitly mentions that although she had always 'supported the idea that the adoptive family and adoptive culture are what mark you for ever … now I do not know what I should believe'.

In her story, we can see the importance of physical resemblance in the recognition of a family identity but also the difficulties of constructing that identity in some of the things that separate her from her biological family.

> They are my people without them really being my people, because there is nothing apart from the physical aspect that joins us … In the little house in Kalgaon-Thadi town I confirm once again that I am an Occidental girl from head to toes in the worst sense of the word. I have been raised with all the comforts and now I would be unable to sleep on the floor of the little living room … together with the others, literally side by side, without any kind of privacy. (Miró 2004: 74–75)

It is interesting to note that, at the same time as she mentions the things that separate her from her biological family, she 'feels at home' and notes that they 'are joined by strong feelings'. But in the end and despite the physical meeting, it is photographs that are the visual confirmation, 'objectified' or '(de)subjectified', of the truth of the relationship through recognition in the body of the other. 'Asha and Savita show me family photos and the two kids also join us, making comments about them. This is the moment that has united us the most since I have arrived … Now I do feel at home, with my family. And they do too' (Miró 2004).

Is Physical Resemblance a Confirmation of the 'Genetic' Facts of Kinship?

Catalan kinship ideas and assumptions show that family resemblance originates in the identity of sharing 'biogenetic substance'. This identity is the main source of the relational aspect of kinship. Here we draw on a statement about physical resemblance made by a woman who painfully remembers an abortion resulting from an amniocentesis test. Francesca is in her mid-forties and lives in a small town in Catalonia. Her family owns a food business that was set up by her father and his brothers. Nowadays, Francesca, together with her sister and her cousins, runs the business. She is married to a man nine years her junior who comes from the same region of Catalonia as her and with whom she has an eight-year-old daughter. She learnt of our research project through a bulletin published by a fertility self-help association and she contacted us to tell us she was happy to be interviewed. During a long interview at her home, Francesca recalled the ultrasound scan, where she could see the fetus but which led to the end of her pregnancy. In her words:

> I could see it so clearly that it seemed to me that it resembled my other daughter … The mouth looked well formed, her hands, every part of her body, the long arms, and the legs. The long arms, like those of my husband's family, and I thought this is going to be a very tall baby and with full lips like those of my daughter, who has protruding lips.

In the memory of the ultrasound scan, she establishes a relationship between the fetus and her daughter and her husband and his family. The fetus becomes a person in her memory through its resemblance with them. It becomes an individual person to the extent that it was being formed through relations of family resemblance. The highly medicalised context in which these images of physical resemblance are shown can lead us to give more credit to biological 'facts' than to social ties. After all, resemblance between these bodies has always been there: it has just been awaiting social acknowlcdgcmcnt. From confirmation of the family resemblance of certain features of the fetus, Francesca builds up ties of social identity between the fetus and her family. The sight of the foetus appears to confirm an obvious truth: children resemble their parents and their siblings – a truth that comes from biological facts. In support of this interpretation, we might include other associations that Francesca made during our conversation. She told us that kids 'resemble the family' and that is due to 'genetics': 'And the generation ... younger than you, you see them ... and they have two or three children. How cute, and they are so beautiful and all alike, similar and part of the family, don't you think so? And that is because it is in the gene, that's it.' Toying with the idea of adopting children, which she considered after two miscarriages, she said she found it difficult because 'you do not see anything resembling you'. This, again, she ascribes to 'genetics'. The image shown by the ultrasound scan is a stimulus to build ties with the fetus on the basis of a family resemblance between it and the family body. The person is being constructed through resemblance relations with members of the family. It is a continuity of these relations. A fetus technologised and geneticised by the ultrasound image is transformed, through the eyes of the mother, into a relational entity; an entity that becomes part of the family body through the knowledge of kinship. Family resemblances are precisely what define family identity.

Maria, another woman, who was preparing herself for an in vitro fertilisation cycle, talked about how curious she was 'to learn what a son born to them was going to be like ... would he resemble him [her husband], or me?' Knowledge of family resemblance creates relations and constitutes a form of recognition of family identity. Through the images of the fetus or through the 'curiosity to learn', physical resemblance constitutes the relational identity of kinship. Knowledge is a way of establishing family identities. For this reason, the affliction over not being able to bear children is expressed as an impossibility to know. As one infertile woman told us: 'It hurts me so much not being able to have a baby with my husband, not being able to see our resemblance to a child born to us.' It is the impossibility of knowing that becomes the source of the affliction. Notice that this knowledge is mainly visual; it has to do with 'seeing'. In this way family resemblance is related to the curiosity to know.

Is this knowledge of kinship related to biogenetic substance, or is it knowledge built around family identity? Despite the fact that 'biological inheritance' (in the words of adoptive parents) or 'the kin in the gene' (in the words of Finkler 2001: 235) is taboo and seldom, if ever, talked about, some of these parents face this matter with anxiety. As Finkler commented in her study of what she calls the medicalisation of kinship, many adoptees and/or their adoptive families share the sentiment that adopted children are not persons because they do not have a medical history (Finkler 2001). To ease their anxiety, some Catalan adoptive families adopt from Haiti because in some orphanages they can meet the biological parents or the child's mother when they go to collect the child. The more information they can give to their children – in response to questions concerning their identity – the more confident the parents are in the success of their task. For many adoptive parents, knowing birth parents can provide more information about the child both in the present and in the future. For many adoptees, to meet their biological parents or relatives is also a means of having more information about themselves. One mother, who narrates her meeting with the biological parents of her two daughters, considered it to be a valuable experience. Seeing them had helped her understand why her girls were so small despite the age that the orphanage declared they were. They were tiny because their parents were tiny and not because they had been ill or undernourished.

The Given Aspect in Adoptive Kinship

Modell has written that, in some cases, previous encounters between adoptive parents and the child provide the first step for matching. Prospective parents meet a particular child 'on paper, online, or in person [and] surface traits strike the chord that begins a movement toward a permanent relationship'. In these contexts matching 'comes to depend upon a spontaneous, unpredictable and personalized response. These responses are not, however, free. They are constrained by expectations about "desirable" children' (Modell 2002: 157). An adoptive mother in Barcelona explained what happened when they had to choose their boy in this way:

> It is a step ... a little bit distressing ... yes ... because it is your first time but once it has been done there are no more problems, are there? ... There were not so many children in the room: a couple of twins ... a boy older than our biological daughter ... and there was S. ... probably some more but ... I do not remember ... My husband immediately took a good look at S., the only boy in that room who was not looking at us, who was doing nothing and who was as if he was hiding.

'He Was Our Child from the Moment We Walked In that Room' is the title of the paper in which Krusiewicz and Wood (2001) analyse the 'magnetism and a quick identification, empathy and pity' (Modell 2002) that many adoptive parents refer to when they describe their first encounter with their child. But this first encounter is not always the origin of a 'movement toward a relationship'. The importance given by adoptive parents to the possibility of identification, or the matching of them with their child, sometimes allows them to justify their rejection of a child because of their difficulty in identifying themselves physically with the child on the first encounter. Referring to this, an adoptive mother recounted the following on an Internet LISTSERV:

> Each person has the strength to face some problems. I remember the case of a couple that adopted in Russia. After their first visit, they rejected a baby on racial grounds. For me it was terrible but they really needed a physical resemblance with the baby so as to identify themselves as parents. They were consistent with their awareness of their own strengths and the child they eventually adopted is perfectly integrated with them and their eldest [biological] daughter.

But in many cases the decision to allocate a child to a family does not depend on the parents: it is a professional decision. When Modell (2002) analysed the role assigned to resemblance in adoption processes in the United States, she pointed out that resemblances are important not only for adoptive parents but also for professionals in charge of adoption processes. For having a child who looks like an adoptive father 'normalizes the adoptive relationship, putting it into the same picture gallery as the biological family' and making it more secure and enduring.

> Social workers take the matter of resemblance seriously, and decisions about an adoption support the adage of blood's thickness. Throughout the twentieth century, the practice of matching dominated placement decision: the baby to be placed in an adoptive home should 'match' the parents in that home. Match in race and in religion, of course, but also in physique, intelligence and temperament. (Modell 2002: 6–7)

But Modell thinks that the practice is changing and being cloaked in another language. She describes it as 'the language of bonding, belonging, and enduring solidarity', which goes from genealogical connections to parental love (Modell 2002: 6–7). Nevertheless, and also probably as proof of a changing time, adoptive parents still believe in the importance of matching procedures and resemblances in adoption processes, including international and interracial adoptions. According to Spanish parents adopting in China, the photographs included in the dossier required by the CCAA (China Centre for Adoption Affairs) when the process of child adoption begins are also used for matching purposes. They are used to match them with the girl who most resembles them. There is an extensive and elaborated narrative about the way matching works in Chinese adoptive processes.

Families who adopt in China call attention to what they call the 'matching room': the place in the CCAA building where many civil servants devote their whole working day to 'matching' applicant families with girls to be adopted. The 'matching room' is, according to adoptive parents, where the placement process finishes. This is a very important fact for them because it is the step immediately before the image of the girl that has been allocated to them is sent to them. According to the stories of Spanish adoptive families, civil servants look for a bond between the girls and their parents and by closely examining the records they must 'match' the photographs in the adoptive families' dossier and the photographs of the girls who come from a number of orphanages. And if there is no physical resemblance, another matching criterion is used. For example, in one case the girl sang softly all the time and they knew that one of the parents liked music. An adoptive mother explained the work of the Chinese civil servants on an Internet LISTSERV as follows:

> They try to match a family with a baby born on a date close to one of the future parents' birthdays or their wedding anniversary, or close to one of the future grandparents' birthdays. They also pay attention to the baby's and parents' interests (for example, music), and to the parents' and baby's faces. I do not know if these matching 'rules' are followed in a predetermined order or not. After all, I believe it is what many people would call 'at random', but some of us believe that those matches are guided by an invisible hand.

The 'matching room' is a place in the CCAA that many families photograph and describe in detail when they go to China, and photographs of it are found not only on Spanish but also North American LISTSERVS and web pages.[1] Narratives about the 'matching rooms' vary but, in general, the most outstanding feature of the people who work there is their carefulness and in particular the time they devote to the 'matching' process. They clearly are thought to have in mind the importance of the task for the future success of the adoption.

The matching room is the place where the first ties take place. In many cases there is an idea of 'predestination', which implies that the child was born with relationships that were waiting for somebody who could find them and give them a social acknowledgement. On the China Internet LISTSERV, one adoptive mother said that she asked a CCAA worker about the process they had developed in the 'matching room' and explained in this way what the CCAA worker replied:

> When it is your agency's turn, the computer starts with the photo of your face (or of the married couple) along with information about the place where you live, your profession, your favourite leisure activity and the age of the girl requested. It is a one-page screen. In the cubicle where you are matched, a woman will have several records of girls (there seemed to be between five and ten girls). The opening page is the very same wonderful page you receive when we get the placement. It has the main photo of the girl. First of all, they pay attention to job and leisure activity to check if there is something in the group that matches those. For example, if you state that you love music and the child's record states that she loves music, the woman could match you. Or if the father is a sports fan and the record of the child states that she is 'very active', they could be matched. Another example I was given is that if somebody says that they love gardening and

the name of the girl means 'little turnip' (hahaha) or something like that, this could be another reason for matching. Sometimes there is no meaningful or somewhat relevant personal information about the parents. In that case, the woman, who has your record, would pick up several photos of children to 'see', as if it were magic, a possible match.

This narrative of an adoptive mother about the activities of women working in the matching room may seem idealised, but it suggests the 'shared creation of family's destiny' (Howell 2003: 467) which, according to Howell, is one of the most important kin-constituting factors. A Chinese girl's grandmother, awaiting her second granddaughter, sent us the photographs of both the girls to break the news that she was going to be a grandmother for the second time. When we received the photos via email, we asked her (via online personal messenger chat) about her new granddaughter, and she explained:

> The Chinese are great because, obviously, in these photos they look like sisters, everybody tells me so. Of course some say: 'sure, all Chinese people look alike'. But it is not true, because in the 'matching room' they look for resemblances between the girls if possible ... and a little resemblance with their parents. If you have a dimple in your cheek, they will look for one in the child's ... Some of them said that A. looked like me because she was chubby and had a round face! And many times, when you see a photo of the girl with her parents, you say: 'gosh, but there is a resemblance ... an expression that is similar ... to the father or to the mother'. This is the reason why, in the list, we always say that the Chinese are great.

Norwegian parents harbour similar notions that staff in the donor country try to match the child they have been given with themselves, but they seem less concerned with this than Spanish couples. Norwegian adoption workers think that it is a response to demands from North American and European adoption agencies. Even if they had an ambition to do something like that, how could they possibly examine the more than 10,000 adoptions that are transacted every year in China? But the point is not whether this kind of matching work takes place or not in China – or elsewhere – but that Spanish couples feel a need for this to be so. The desire for the existence of a matching room such as the one in Beijing is in itself an interesting fact. When prospective parents embark upon the process of adopting a child from an alien country, they activate a biological model by employing terms like pregnancy and birth (Howell and Marre, 2006).

As we saw with Francesca, when she painfully remembered her miscarriage resulting from the amniocentesis test, in international adoptions in China the 'kinning' process starts when parents begin, by themselves or through the decisions of professionals or civil servants, to transform a child's image into a relational entity that becomes a family body through the knowledge of kinship.

Building Kinship through Children's Images in International Adoption

Adoptive parents also referred to the 'truth given by an image of the child' as a way to become more confident in their decision and, also, to begin to build ties – or what Howell calls the 'kinning' process (Howell 2003). Cartwright (2003) remarks that images, visual media and child portrait photographs are at the centre of the culture of international adoption. In some countries, including the United States, agencies circulate images of children available for adoption through web pages, computer databanks and brochures 'with surprising ease' (Cartwright 2003: 83). In many of these cases, the images of 'awaiting children' are completed with some biographical and/or medical data. In many cases, the images of awaiting children also serve as tools in medical screening and for the evaluation of possible pathologies according to which children might be accepted or rejected. Cartwright notes that interpreting casual portraits by looking for medical information has become a common practice in international adoption. One specific example is the screening of the child portrait for fetal alcohol syndrome (FAS). In this case, the image functions somewhat like data from a prenatal test. It is a medical technique that is beset with the historical problem of pathologising signifiers of cultural difference (Cartwright 2003: 83–84). Despite the fact that much research on adoption is concerned with forms of adaptation in general and the adjustment of adoptees in particular, the 'kinning' process begins before the children arrive home. The process begins at 'birth', when parents receive the first evidence of what their child will be like. This usually takes the form of a small image sent by the institution in charge of the adoption process in the child's country of origin. Adoptive parents arrive at the end of the 'bureaucratic pregnancy', in their words, when they know 'their' child and when they receive the first images. These images, which many families quickly share with the international adoption's cyber community, become 'an object with which an unbreakable bond can be forged' and that is 'the promise of exchange for the original' (Anagnost 2000: 406).

At this time, adoptive families concentrate on the kin relationship they can build or would like to build with their adoptive children. On the child's image, an image with no body, as Telfer (1999) puts it, parents begin to build kin relationships by looking for family resemblances that allow them to forge family continuities and identities. Having and looking at the photograph of the adopted child establish an immediate tie. The act of looking at the photograph turns the isolated and far-off body of the image into a relational person who has a context within which they can develop a relationship. In this sense, for some adoptive parents that first image becomes 'a coveted family photograph, representing an imagined future family member much as a foetal sonogram might do' (Cartwright 2003: 84).

In her essay on the 'imaginary body', Stewart (1993) gives singular importance to family images. For her, it is a 'technology capable of completing the subjective identification between parent and child, a technology that is contemporaneous with the intensification of family life in its modern form' (Anagnost 2000: 406, 419 citing Stewart 1993). Image practices that Telfer (1999) mentions provide opportunities to interrogate the cultural potency of corporeal resemblance and connectedness. The image becomes the icon of a future relation and by abduction (Peirce 1965) it makes an imagined kin relationship real. From then on, the relationship becomes concrete and the identity of the child can develop on concrete knowledge. Imaginary relatedness becomes a real relationship. As in biological forms of pregnancy and birth, including the ones linked to new reproductive technologies (NRT), the images also function in helping parents to imagine 'their' child or themselves as parents of children 'like these'.

Krusiewicz and Wood (2001) analysed eighteen parents' 'entrance stories'. They understood 'entrance stories' as the accounts of how and why a particular child became part of a particular family. They categorised recurrent themes in five principal ways: dialectical tensions, destiny and compelling connection (which occurred forty-eight, forty-five and forty-eight times, respectively) and rescue and legitimacy twenty-six and thirty-two occurrences). Amongst the most common theme under 'compelling connections' was physical connection through appearance (Krusiewicz and Wood 2001: 795). Following Hoffman-Reim (1990), the authors point out that 'through the similarity of physical appearance, habits, or personality traits, the construction of resemblance allows persons to move closer together'. In different ways, either through celebrating physical resemblance or acknowledging the lack of it, a compelling connection between parents and children is highlighted. Participants also portrayed a connection so compelling that it compensated for the fact that their children did not 'grow in their tummies' (Krusiewicz and Wood 2001: 795).

A person 'naturalises' the adoption process through identifying him/herself with the adopted child by looking for some elements that establish resemblance between the adopted child and the adopting person or family. A woman who adopted in Haiti told us:

> when I was confirmed the adoption and received the photo, I sent it to my mother by email. My old woman was phoning me up every ten minutes the whole afternoon. I think she would look at the photo and phone again. And she told me this girl looks exactly like you. Yes, that is what your hair looked like when you were a child.

The resemblance, concludes this woman, is something intrinsic to families; they form their identity through resemblance. 'In those families with adopted children you see them alike, maybe it has to do with gestures rather than features, but ... they end up being alike.'

Final Remarks

Through family resemblance, connection and recognition are constructed between relatives. It is a way of thinking about the continuity between bodies – a body that, within Western tradition, is not clearly delimited by biological inheritance. How can we explain family resemblance – the relational aspect of a person – and at the same time the idiosyncrasy and diversity of human beings – the individual aspect of a person? Pliny (1969: 51–54) explained it by means of the fortuitous circumstances of the moment of conception and the higher cognitive speed of man compared with animals:

> Family resemblance cases are an extremely broad issue and include many fortuitous circumstances – visual and auditory memories and images perceived in the moment of conception. A thought that suddenly pops up in the mind of one of the parents is supposed to produce resemblance or to cause a mixture of characteristics. And the reason why there are more differences in man than in other animals is that the thinking speed, mood quickness and wit diversity print multiform models. In other animals, on the contrary, their minds are motionless and they are identical to one another of the same gender.

It is noticeable that these kinds of resemblances, brought about in the moment of conception, are also found in Portugal (Pina-Cabral 2002) and Panama (Gudeman 1976). So, using these ideas about the influence of the circumstances and of the mind on the conception and development of a body as a starting point, we can understand traditional rituals and beliefs we find in Europe concerning conception, pregnancy, birth and the first days of the newborn baby. Cultural perceptions search for a way to establish identity through resemblances between bodies and mimesis is a key element in the construction of the body. In this case, the body is subjected to both physical and moral inheritance – the structural aspect of kinship – and, at the same time, to circumstances and events – the fortuitous aspect of kinship. According to our knowledge about genetic inheritance, variability is in the genes – not in external circumstances and even less in the human mind. Nevertheless, when we wonder about the continuity between bodies in contexts where there is a clear genetic discontinuity – as is the case of gamete donation or transnational adoption – physical resemblance reappears as a way of recognising identity.

We must bear in mind that, despite the fact that assisted reproduction techniques favour biological descendants, our informants did not express a radical opposition between biological and adopted children. Gamete donations imply some kind of mediating gradation between the two opposite poles. In any case, the choice of assisted reproduction techniques is based on the uncertainty of biological reproduction, while adoption is based on the certainty of social filiation. In this context, we could say that there is a radical displacement of the usual order of kinship: in opposition to the traditional understanding of kinship, here nature becomes uncertain and 'adoptive' kinship becomes the most certain. Nevertheless, kinship allows the constant change from the natural to the social without the need of setting one of them as determining or dominant. That is why there is no contradiction between wanting to adopt and wanting a biological child. Family identity is constructed through both the knowledge of gametes and genetic inheritance and affective ties developed between relatives.

Legal and medical concepts on assisted reproduction tend to prioritise the individualistic and biological aspects – donor anonymity, genetic information, the status of the embryo and so on. These are aspects that establish an empty space in connection with the relational elements of kinship. On the contrary, the insistence on resemblance as a key element in the construction of the family body proves the presence of a relational concept of the person. We have argued that the relational aspect of the individual person is connected with the 'given' aspect of kinship. It has been conceptualised as the natural aspect of kinship – sharing bio-genetic substances – but it is clearly related to ideas of identification that adoptive parents see in the image of their adopted children.

In adoption processes where there is no common biogenetic substance and adoption is legally defined as a substitute for 'natural' descent, the presence of bodily images of children put up for adoption and the constitution of resemblances with them show the extent that knowledge of kinship, through resemblance, is necessary to construct family identity. This is an issue that goes beyond the constitution of a person as an individual based on a set of genes or as an issue revolving exclusively around origins. Catalan adoptive parents also consider resemblance as a way of strengthening connections. They 'transubstantiate' their identity in the body of the adopted child by establishing resemblance, by naming and by identifying the typical behaviour of the family body. While resemblance is not always physical, it always has positive functions. We can still take from Freud's definition of identification the idea that the child always identifies himself or herself with the beloved person.

Note

1. http://www.angelcovers.org/ccaaset2.shtml; http://www.familyoffour.homestead.com/June05CCAA.html. Another way in which the 'matching room' is described in the adoptive families in China's' LISTSERV is also interesting:

    On your right, you can see stacks of dossiers. There are ten of them, with six each. On your left, there is a cabinet with information about all the girls. In the middle, there is a table for the people. I believe that I have only seen women working there. There must be fifteen of them, separated by little folding screens, so that they can concentrate, I guess. It is a room with natural light. You get there through a long hall with the other CCAA Departments on both sides. And at the end of it, two steps up, you find the matching room.

CHAPTER 5

THE CONTRIBUTION OF HOMOPARENTAL FAMILIES TO THE CURRENT DEBATE ON KINSHIP

Anne Cadoret

How do people become a family today? Who will be assigned the term 'parent' when we consider adoptive families, people who have recourse to medically assisted reproduction, reconstituted families or homoparental families?[1] In Western societies kinship has traditionally been based on the coincidence of social kinship and biological kinship. This led us to believe that knowledge of the biological would provide the ultimate explanation for kinship, since the parents were the genitors and there are only two parents: a father and a mother. The construction of kinship could be described but it could not be questioned. Subsequently, with advances in biological understandings of procreation concurrent with new family configurations and new possibilities for dissociating sexuality and procreation, the construction of the family has become increasingly complicated: the two genitors are no longer automatically the parents of the child, since kinship does not always emanate from their bodies. Furthermore, the body of the mother and the body of the father do not contribute in the same way to the production of the child and the reproduction of the family.

Researchers have recently shown a renewed interest in studying kinship. At the dawn of the twenty-first century, they are asking how these two different forms of kinship, the biological and the social, are combined into the same family unit. Can kinship still be called natural? If not, how should the old nature-culture debate be posed? How can the truth about Western kinship be discovered? Or, rather, we could ask: What are the ground rules for establishing the truth of Western kinship? Is it a truth object resting on a single gene or is it, on the contrary, a personal truth, bound up with a family or a situation and drawing on several different elements?

Following a review of the terms of the debate and the impossibility of a nature without a culture, that is to say, without a concurrent symbolic interpretation of the human body, I shall examine how homoparental lesbian families, having recourse to donor insemination, are able to 'make a family' and how they deal with the distinction between production and reproduction that is at the very core of their parental couple. The ways in which they create a family and the name of the father which they decide to give or not to give to the genitor seems to me to bring into focus questions that allow us to move forward in the current debate on the construction of kinship.

The Body Cannot Be Reduced to the Biological: Nature Is Always Cultural

The Empire of the Biological

For some fifteen years now, Western kinship has re-emerged as a central issue debated by anthropologists, as seen in the numerous recent works on this topic.[2] Schneider argued for the biological anchoring of Western kinship. In his words, '[k]inship is whatever the biogenetic relationship is. If science discovers new facts about biogenetic relationship, then that is what kinship is and was all along, although it may not have been known at that time' (Schneider 1968: 23).[3] Here he was attacking anthropologists' ethnocentrism and charging them with looking at the societies they studied through the prism of their own Western culture and using tools appropriate for Western societies but inadequate for non-Western societies.[4] Yet I believe that Schneider did not bring his critique to its logical conclusion, that he did not properly analyse the roots of this ethnocentrism, thus failing to unravel – to deconstruct – Western kinship. He did not attempt to understand 'kinship in the making'. True, he showed that the American system of kinship in the 1950s and 1960s (more specifically among middle-class whites) based 'good kinship' on biology, in other words transforming genitors into parents, into mother and fathers, duly married to each other. But he did not look into the reasons for basing kinship on biology and took this reduction of kinship to biology as a primary truth entrenched in dogma (Cadoret 2005).[5] In his article 'Virgin Birth', Leach described well how all societies, Western as much as any other, elaborate various beliefs about kinship that lie outside the logic of production and are founded on other symbolic principles: 'If we put the so-called primitive beliefs alongside the sophisticated ones and treat the whole lot with equal philosophical respect we shall see that they constitute a set of variations around a common structural theme, the metaphysical topography of the relationship between gods and men' (Leach 1969: 86). This suggests to me that researchers therefore need to consider what 'metaphysical topography' is being proposed when kinship is based on biological truth.

Production and Reproduction: the First Distinction

This dilution of kinship into another domain of knowledge where kinship becomes the ultimate instance of the recognition of purely biological relationships might explain anthropologists' lack of interest, at least for a period of time, in Western kinship. However, there is also renewed interest resulting from advances in scientific knowledge and reproductive technologies, with respect first, to contraception and secondly, to medically assisted reproduction. The first of these technical advances, contraception, has contributed to the emancipation of women from child bearing ('I'll have a child when and if I want one'), which has gone hand in hand with greater occupational autonomy and new ways of looking at and responding to family life. The second, medically assisted reproduction, has severed the link completely between sexuality and procreation. Sexuality without procreation had already been possible with contraception, and now, with medically assisted reproduction, procreation without sexuality also became possible.

This rupture has resulted in cutting the Gordian knot between sexuality, reproduction, alliance and filiation, and it generates a number of questions about the founding truth constituting the family. Is it a matter of desire, subject therefore to the whims of the individual and her or his personal history? Or is it a matter for legislation, depending on human and political decisions? Or is it, rather, human biological materials that are recognised as the prerequisite to the existence of society? Should all three of these requirements be satisfied to establish filiation, or does one of them take precedence over the other two? What importance should be assigned to procreation in constituting the individual? But also what importance should be given to procreation in constituting kinship?

Production and Reproduction: the Second Distinction

The old nature-culture debate has resurfaced with the concept of 'nature' shifting to first biology and then genes, with both these terms usually used in their adjectival form: the 'biological' and the 'genetic'. Studying the 'nature' of Western kinship has reverted to studying its biological anchorage and the way in which it is achieved, in order to reveal the symbolic order that underlies it. For example, Yanagisako and Collier (1987) raise questions about the Lévi-Straussian 'atom of kinship' depicting the two sexes: 'The standard units of our genealogies, after all, are circles and triangles about which we assume a number of things. Above all, we take for granted that they represent two naturally different categories of people and that the natural difference between them is the basis for human reproduction and, therefore, kinship' (Yanagisako and Collier 1987: 32). With this remark about the naturalisation of kinship in two sexes, these authors criticise the naturalisation of male domination without, however, challenging the consequences of the role of and control by biological knowledge with respect to the very determination of the kinship relations.[6] These questions arise in conjunction with the renewed distinction between production and reproduction. Here we see Strathern (1995) dissociating productive kinship, anchored in biology and the various manipulations of human reproduction such as genetic modification, from the reproduction of kinship. The former, productive kinship, gives the embryo which is made up of its genetic substances an individuality; and the latter, re-production, refers to starting over again. As Strathern reminds us: 'Reproduction commonly means to bring into existence something that already exists in another form' (1995: 354). Reproduction has several meanings: in addition to making a copy or making anew, it also means to recall something – it involves the daily task of working on existing elements and of making existing elements one's own.

Strathern, in the same article, attempts to make sense of the consequences of new reproductive technologies for the production/reproduction dichotomy within Western contexts. For some time, the production and reproduction of children were distributed between the same actors, that is, the mother and father within the family unit (the form studied by Schneider); both the mother and the father were responsible for the production and reproduction of the child.

But the changes over time in family configurations, together with an increasing number of adoptions, reconstituted families and medically assisted reproduction, seriously dented the coincidence of creating and reproducing children. The child's genitors are no longer necessarily its parents. Today, '[d]ispersed kinship is constituted in dispersed conception; it includes those who "produce" the child with assistance as well as those who assist. As a consequence, there thus exists a field of procreators whose relationship to one another and to the product of conception is contained in the act of conception itself and not in the family as such' (Strathern 1995: 352). The whole debate from now on hinges on the ties between the producers and reproducers of children, as well as between the producers and the children themselves. As Strathern notes, 'Procreation creates a kinship that was formed first and foremost in biogenetic relations' (ibid.). First, I would like to point out that this relationship is only biogenetic and that it is relevant here to question how it is known. Strathern emphasises the autonomy of genes relative to their donors and the personality of the donors, and that the more science enables us to fully comprehend genes or the genome, the less it becomes necessary to determine the relationship with donors: 'The more knowledge Euro-Americans have of the likelihood of disorders being transmitted and the more accurate the tracing of genetic components, the less necessary it becomes to know the identity of the parent. More kinship, fewer relatives' (Strathern 1995: 356–57).

The Odour of Kinship

What does this break between production and reproduction mean? If there is a rupture, can we still talk of kinship? I remain intrigued by how these are used with respect to kinship – as applied by Strathern above. What precisely is the nature of the ties? What do they contain? Is it the 'odour of kinship', of which Pierre Damien already spoke in the eleventh century – an 'odour of kinship' that rules out marriage between individuals already closely related to each other in order to allow their marriage as soon as this kith and kin link disappears, in other words, as soon as these individuals feel they do not belong to the same circle of close relatives? Françoise Héritier quotes Pierre Damien who wrote in the eleventh century: 'There, where the hand of kinship is absent, which brought together those whom it caught in its web, marriage throws out its fishing hook to draw in those who are further away' (Héritier 1981: 150, (literally translated by Bolland)).[7] In short, where kinship fails, marriage is there to bring back those who stray. The 'kinship odour' does not so much reveal a person's identity but mostly organises social exchange through matrimonial exchange, that is to say, designates those who can get married and those who can't. This then becomes a matter of elaborating the social bond of alliance through a representation of the body and by choosing the significant substances that will define the person and his or her ancestors attached within. In a way, one's relatives are personified in the body by the bond of blood.

It seems interesting to me to consider how 'kinship odour' is constituted. Is it limited to knowledge of how biological reproduction occurs, as a reductionist explanation would have us believe? Or does it include from the start, once it is detected, many other elements, some of which are also bodily (such as cytoplasm), while others are social and symbolic? As a function of the way in which the social and symbolic order is constructed, each culture selects what it considers as significant substances (see Héritier 1977). We become aware that if '[r]eproduction commonly means to bring into existence something that already exists in another form', to recall Strathern's formulation, which I quoted earlier, then the spoken word and the symbolic are also required to enable the passage from one form to the other, that is, from production to reproduction. Yet, in Strathern's formulation, this transfer takes place without any explanation. I see in this metamorphosis – the conversion of production into re-production – a conjuring trick, for one has to displace (or should we say 'replace'?) the other and in so doing reproduction conceals production.

Filiation Truth

Since the Enlightenment, Western culture has trained us to look for scientific truth in every natural fact, to disentangle the elements to reach the hard kernel of this fact, thereby making it incontestable. The gene, today the determining element of production of the body, falls under this type of truth, at least in some popular representations. It seems to me important to question how we use this scientific truth, and I ask myself the following question: when it comes to knowing our own kinship, what gives us the certainty of the truth about our genes? In his analysis of regimes of truth, Foucault distinguishes between two forms of truth: one he called 'event truth' (*vérité-événement*) and the other 'demonstration truth' (*vérité-démonstration*); one is specific to a place, a person, a particular moment in time; the other is a universal claim. Purveyors of the first truth 'are those who hold the secrets of a place, those who have spoken the requisite words and made the ritual gestures, those whom the truth has chosen to enlighten: the prophets, the divinities, the innocent, the blind, the mad, the wise, etc.' (Foucault 2003: 237 (translated by Bolland)).[8] This event truth does not so much come from the domain of truth as we understand it today as from the charismatic power of its proponents, who were able to impose 'their truth' through the strength of their own convictions, proof of which was made, for example, through ordeals by fire. Meanwhile, the second regime of truth depends on negotiation, demonstration and knowledge of the object, and no longer involves knowledge of the self – even if intermediaries are needed to gain access to such knowledge, intermediaries such as doctors and geneticists, specific individuals possessing this knowledge and the scientific techniques to construct this knowledge.

But why is it that this knowledge of our genes (the gene object), this particular truth, should become our truth about the human person? Why would our knowledge of the identity of the gene lead us to the identity of the self? Would we not in fact be making the production of the body and the reproduction of an individual the same thing, thereby passing off truth about an object as truth about the person?

So why, when dealing with filiation, should there be a truth about the body which should stand alone as the truth about kinship? Should there be, within this same body, a substance, a specific particle – the gene – which would be the natural and immutable root of the body and the foundation of kinship? In the light of the advances in knowledge about procreation, do we have to accept that the gene should become the very substance, the kernel to which our intellectual search would be restricted and which would lead us to define kinship? My parents, my father, my mother – are they my genitors? Or, rather, are they only my genitors? Or, even, do my genitors necessarily have to be my parents? Should kinship be defined by the act of procreation, by the sheer production of the child?

Yet the exercise of parenting is not restricted to procreation, but also entails other tasks just as necessary as birth in the construction of the human person: activities such as feeding the child, rearing it, providing a name, transmitting status. These are tasks which our society assigns to persons considered to be the genitors. I see in this assignment a further conjuring trick of transforming production into reproduction and thereby hiding reproduction behind the curtain of production, in the fact that a child has a father and a mother and above all a single father and a single mother. This assignment is made through our rules of filiation: the child has to have two parents who provide him or her with a family name and first names, who have parental authority and who introduce the child into each of their lineages. This assignment is transmitted through the different forms families can take, such as adoptive families (in which the parents replace the genitors), families having recourse to artificial insemination with an anonymous donor (in which the social father is permitted to be considered like the genitor) or, and of particular interest here, homoparental families. In some of these family types, the parents may still pose themselves as possible genitors of their children, and, in such permutations, the filiative fiction may still work; however, this is not possible in the case of homoparental families. Two parents of the same sex are not able, between themselves only, to produce a child and pretend they are the genitors. Homoparental families cannot imitate a family consisting only of a father, a mother and their children. They seem to me to be interesting to 'dissect', for they provide situations of reproduction that necessarily reveal the way in which kinship is social.

We should first point out that homoparental families are conjugated in the plural, some preferring to construct themselves by a general reference to a father and a mother and opting for co-parenting: a man and a woman, typically a gay and a lesbian, each of them usually living in a homosexual couple, agree to have a child together and to become legally the father and mother, while living in separate households. While this configuration has similarities with a reconstituted family, the child, if he or she has a father and mother, as in heteroparental families, nearly always also has two maternal figures and two paternal figures, for which the reference model of a single-father and single-mother family becomes totally inadequate.[9] Other homosexual parents prefer the stability of the single domestic household for their child and do not want their conjugal couple to be disturbed by another parent: therefore they are inclined towards adoption or medically assisted reproduction. Yet their status as a homosexual couple precludes them from benefiting from either of these two channels to parenthood in France: they either remain silent about their homosexuality and their affective life (if they are applying to social services for adoption), or they go abroad to avail themselves of medically-assisted reproduction.[10] With their single status, homoparental families in domestic units cannot be assimilated as genitors when they adopt, or as parents when they choose artificial insemination. The child's production is no longer convertible into the family's reproduction; implicitly they have sexuality (they live together) but not procreative sexuality. For the first time, we are dealing with a new symbolic order where sexuality will never be procreative but always for pleasure only.

Making Kinship

Depending on the type of family they have constructed, homosexual parents will have to answer different questions about assigning familial status to each member of the couple. For example, those who opt for co-parenting do not have to differentiate the genitors from the parents, since the genitors are also the parents; however, they will generally share their parental functions with their same-sex partner, who may also claim the status of parent. Their efforts to construct a family will then consist in establishing a multiple-parent arrangement, as well as getting legal recognition of the family unit. It is no longer a question of the configuration of the two-parent family but of three- or even four-parent families.[11] Those who choose adoption find themselves by definition in a situation of social kinship – reproduction, even if such reproduction in the framework of a homoparental family is still difficult and quite poorly recognised. Regarding women who avail themselves of medically assisted reproduction, they have to form a family of two persons of the same sex of which one is the social, legal and biological mother of the child; they will have to create a place for the female partner of the biological mother, as well as to decide the place of the absent genitor – the sperm donor. If the reproduction of the child is so visibly detached from its production for one of the parents but not for the other, how are reproduction and production to be constructed and articulated? What, for instance, did Isabelle and Maria (two informants I met during my fieldwork) do to make a family?[12]

I shall retrace the major stages of their process of 'making kinship', since their story is exemplary of the way family reproduction works. We can observe how families are constructed in this society by following, in my example, how each woman became a parent, both in her daily life and in the way they talked about it and the explanations they provided. Their story – evolving from two people in love with each other to a family with three children and the parents consisting of the two women – can be separated into two main parts: first, the forming of the couple and the arrival of their children, and second, the symbolic assertion of the existence of each parental lineage as well as legal recognition in so far as legislation permits. The first part corresponds to the phase of child production, the second to the phase of reproduction within a particular family framework.

Creating the Family Unit and Conception of the Child

Isabelle and Maria met when they were both fourteen years old and together at the same secondary school in Paris. Isabelle was part of an extended family, with numerous brothers and sisters, but also uncles, aunts, grandparents: a family where the table was always ready for friends. Maria, whose Italian father and American mother lived an artist's life in Paris, was a single child.

They fell in love with each other quite rapidly with this adolescent love being the first of other encounters. Maria made the acquaintance of a man, Léon, whom she brought to Isabelle's home several times and the duo, Maria and Léon, uneventfully became a trio, Maria, Léon and Isabelle. Isabelle recalled these times (the 1980s) as 'very pleasant years, cool. Maria passed half her time with Léon and the other half with me. Then it got hard for Maria to choose and Léon didn't want our time to be shared like this any more. So we lived together.' As for Maria, she found it difficult to choose and 'I've got to say that since I was fourteen years old, I've always been the friend of the family and for family parties, like birthdays, at Isabelle's home, Léon and I were invited; then, when Isabelle became part of our couple, it all worked very naturally'.

When, a few years later, after our two friends had left Léon, the question arose of making a family and, fortified by their experience of a 'three-person couple', they both thought of creating a family like the one they had just known, with a man that both of them would love and with whom they would have a child: 'We were sure we would meet another man who we'd fall in love with again; and then it would all happen. A love story with the three of us, with one child, two children, three children.' At this point in their story, having a child meant having a continuous and open relationship with a man, filiation being combined with heterosexual alliance (marriage or co habitation): a child lives with a father and a mother – why not two mothers?

In 1985 they made the acquaintance of another man, Paul, who was himself also homosexual and who had lived for a time in the United States with his partner, Bill. The two had returned to France, in Paul's case for work, Bill for health reasons. This friendship with Paul, which had begun before he left for the United States, transformed itself into a very strong four-way friendship, 'a bit like a couple experiencing love at first sight'. But Bill was increasingly developing the symptoms of Aids: medication was expensive and he didn't have medical coverage in France. Friendship meant showing solidarity, and Isabelle, unquestionably French, married Bill, giving him access to free health care. Maria and Paul were the witnesses at their marriage. There was not a big celebration 'because, anyway, it wasn't a marriage'; they just informed their close kin – brothers, sisters, the mother, for example – about the change in their situation. Bill died and Isabelle became a widow. The possibility of having a child, which could have been envisaged in the framework of this fine four-way friendship, had to be thought of differently: Maria and Isabelle were no longer living with a man with whom they would have a child but, still clinging to the reference model (a child has a father and a mother), they thought for some time about co-parenting[13] and discussed this with two of their male acquaintances who were good friends and 'whom we'd known for ten years, and whom we'd been really very close to', but this project never came to anything. Marie and Isabelle ruled out adoption because access to such kinship was only authorised for a single unit: a duly married couple or a single person. To apply for adoption, our informants would be obliged to present themselves, either one or the other but not both together, to social services as single, and thereby hiding their shared agreement that both of them would become mothers of their children: they refused to lie in this way.

Now their only remaining option was artificial insemination with a donor. This was in 1991–92 and the French bioethics legislation regulating medically assisted reproduction had not yet been adopted (this would happen in 1994) and our informants were able to ask their gynaecologist directly for this procedure. Their gynaecologist chose a donor for them whose identity would remain unknown. The question also arose of 'the mother's womb': which of them, Isabelle or Maria, would start the insemination process and open the way to filiation? They were of the same age and could not take their respective body maturation into account as a criterion for making their decision; so to resolve this they based their decision on the argument of how many descendants there were in their respective families. Isabelle came from a very large family and her brothers and sisters had already provided their parents with grandchildren, while Maria was a single child, so the task fell upon Maria to continue her lineage and become a mother. But the preliminary tests for insemination were negative. Maria was sterile, so Isabelle took over and had a child. As for their next two children, they could no longer appeal to the same doctor since the subsequent bioethics legislation no longer permitted this kind of private agreement and they had to go abroad for Isabelle to be inseminated. They chose Belgium.

We see that Maria and Isabelle had first tried to deal with the question of production by combining production and reproduction in the same family configuration and by thinking of co-parenting. It was only when this solution failed that they turned towards a (relative) dissociation between the two aspects.

Reference to a Cognatic Model: How It Was Symbolically Constructed

Both Maria and Isabelle wanted to be mothers and parents. I shall not elaborate on the sharing of daily domestic and child-rearing tasks, except to point out that, when their children were still very young, they chose to place them in a family-based infant day-care centre (a *crèche parentale*), which meant that one or other of them participated as required in the nursery activities, thereby making their double maternal parenting visible to others.[14] I shall now turn to the role that naming their children played in affirming their kinship and, I shall analyse three dimensions of their naming strategy: the 'family' name, the first names of the children and the terms of address used by the children to refer to each of their parents.

The question of family names and first names allows us to see how the constraints of assigning names are used to affirm a genealogical choice. Freedom of choice in selecting a family name did not exist in France until very recently, the law was unequivocal on the assignment of the family name: children born of married parents took their father's name.[15] However, at the request of one parent or the other, or by the child when he or she reached the age of majority, it was possible to add the name of the mother for private use only. As for a child of unmarried parents, he or she took the father's name if the child was acknowledged simultaneously by both parents, or the mother's name if the mother recognised the child before the father or if only the mother recognised the child. In the case of Isabelle and Maria, whose coupledom was not legally sanctioned, Isabelle was considered to be an unmarried mother and only her family name had been given to the children.[16] But, in practice, for registering in a day-care facility or at school, for example, the two women insisted that both their names be used, thus appropriating for themselves the use of a double name: their daughters carry the family name of Isabelle, their legal mother, and also the family name of Maria. The two mothers asserted their agreement and parental sharing through this first aspect of naming.

Compared with the legal constraints on assigning family names, there is complete freedom in the choice of first names.[17] All the same, this freedom is circumscribed within customs of transmission with parents often assigning to their children the name of one of their kin (a grandparent, brother or sister, godfather, godmother) from one or other of the lineage. Isabelle and Maria chose three names for each of their daughters: the first, Italian-sounding, was a matter of taste and yet it could also be interpreted as the only legal parent, the French mother, paying her respects to the other unofficial parent, the Italian mother; the second and third names, on the other hand, recalled the lineages of both mothers: Claudia, the oldest daughter, was given the name of Maria's grandmother as her second name, and that of Isabelle's great-grandmother as her third; Sofia had the names of Isabelle's deceased husband ('Billy') and Maria's grandfather; finally, Lucia's two last given names are those of Maria's mother and a great-aunt of Isabelle. All these names were consciously chosen so that each of the girls would reflect the two lineages and the diversity of their origins: 'The first given name is Italian, the second American and the third French' (see Figure 5.1). We might therefore ask if these two women situate themselves even more strongly in the traditional schema of lineage perpetuation and the transmission of given names because their own family schema is quite atypical.

As for terms of address, these would also play on the diversity of the origins of both Isabelle and Maria: they are both 'mums', but in two languages, thereby still retaining their individuality: one is called Maman and the other Mamita.

Yet it was painful for Isabelle, the sole legitimate mother, not to have the maternal role of Maria legally recognised. She therefore arranged a 'simple' adoption. This is a complex legal process that involved retaining her kinship relation, but dissociating it from parenting: parental rights and the exercise of the parental role were to be transferred to Maria, with

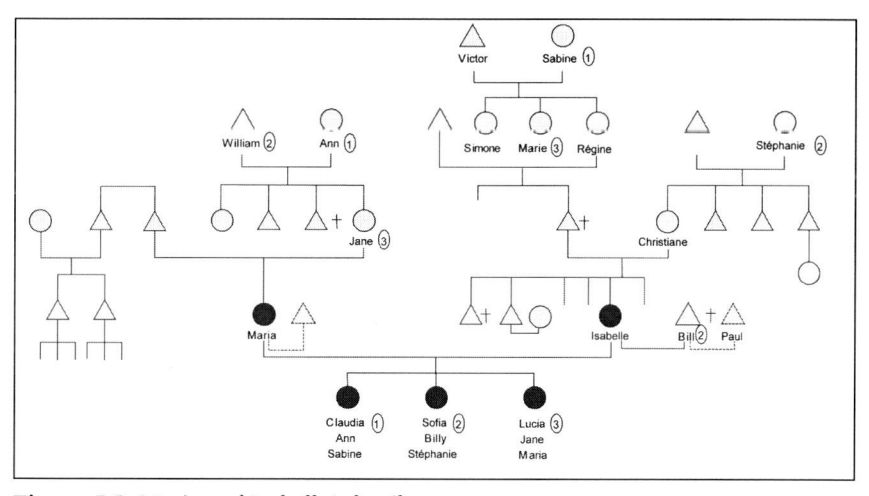

Figure 5.1. Maria and Isabelle's family

Isabelle retaining only her status of ascendant (mother) and losing her parental authority. The children would then officially have the names of both mothers. Finally, three years later, Isabelle regained this parental authority under the new legislation on shared parental rights.[18]

Isabelle and Maria had 'made a family': they adapted the undifferentiated filiation of French society to fit their own needs, and used this as the foundation of their own reproduction, thereby also staking a claim to their own familial identity.[19] The issue of the production of children in the reproduction arrangement remained in question. Isabelle was clearly the genitrix, but what place was to be assigned to the genitor – recognising that this place often combines, either in fiction or in reality, that of the husband or partner of the mother and that of the father of the children?

The Question of 'Genetic Kinship'

Even though my informants claimed they each had equal parental status, they wanted all of their three daughters to have equal filiative status. To achieve this they were to introduce 'the father'. Isabelle and Maria did not dispute that in order to produce a child there had to be an encounter between male and females gametes to make the body and if there was no father who could have been the husband or partner of the mother, 'there had to be someone to replace him'. They wanted to make a family by assigning a place to the sperm donor. First, they gave the same paternity criterion to each of their daughters, basing this on the status of father/donor: since they had not been able to use the same channels for artificial insemination and obtain sperm from the same donor for the first two daughters, they had different 'fathers'; our informants were to maintain the same distinction between their second and third children; although the insemination occurred in the same hospital and it would have been possible to obtain sperm from the same donor, they asked for a different donor.[20] In this way, all three of the girls had the same paternal filiative status, that is, 'unknown filiation', with each of them having their own donor. It is important to note that this identical origin – or, rather, equivalence in its non-identical origin – does not reside in the person of the father but in the reference process, in the intellectual conceptualisation.

There was still the question of paternity to be resolved in the construction of this particular family: paternity in the sense that, according to Marie and Isabelle, 'there had to be someone in his place' – someone whom the children would identify by using the word father but not just the donor of sperm, an abstract, impersonal, corporeal substance. Thus, when a child was asked to draw a family tree and wanted to include her two mothers as her parents, Marie and Isabelle suggested adding a third person: 'If you like, you can put in "papa unknown", because he also exists.' Without realising it, they were adapting to their own situation the critique of Yanagisako and Collier on the representation of the atom of kinship, which, drawn as a circle and a triangle, gives the impression that only a man and a woman can be a mother and father.

I wondered if it was easier for my informants to give the genitor the name of father since the genitor was unknown and could not be called upon to play the material role of the father, by contrast with another informant, Amélie, who categorically refused to use the term father in referring to donors. Unlike Isabelle and Maria, Amélie was living in a family configuration involving artificial insemination with a donor who was known. Moreover, her brother, sensitive to the difficulty lesbians have in becoming mothers, said: 'Yes, I understand. You lesbians have problems [in finding a sperm donor]. So, well, I'm quite ready to become a donor, some day.'[21] He agreed to provide the sperm for two of his sister's lesbian friends, while insisting that he would not become the father of their children. He was himself married and had two children. Amélie, encouraged by her brother's experience, maintained the two terms – genitor and father – each mirroring a different position to be respected in order not to lose the anchor between parents and non-parents.

Our kinship is founded on the idea of a bodily continuity between the mother, the father and their children; this is the basis for wider kinship relations. When artificial insemination is used corporeal continuity cannot substitute itself for the kinship relationship: the donor must not become the father figure.[22] When his identity is known, confusion can easily arise, as Amélie found in the way her mother reacted. Her mother was aware of what her son was doing: 'We didn't want to tell my mother, but she found out about it by chance. She was there the very day these two friends first visited my brother and his wife.' Amélie told us, recognising that this put her mother in an awkward family position. Her mother would become the grandmother of children with whom she would have no biological relationship (the children of Amélie and her female partner), and have no kinship relation with the two other children whom her son produced. This woman, moreover, was present, again by chance, at the rare meetings between Amélie and her two female friends and noticed the physical resemblances between her son (the sperm donor) and the two children. Could this biological relationship become an issue in family inheritance? This is what this biological but non-legal grandmother feared when she telephoned her daughter after one of these encounters to tell her about what she was worried about: 'But, you don't understand, these children will come and claim their part of the inheritance.' The object truth, the truth of the gene, would become the filiation truth. Yet the truth about filiation takes precedence over the object truth; it is not a universal truth, independent of the actual members in the family, but true only when applied to particular families and a particular family constellation. In the construction of Amélie's family, the donor cannot be named father as he is known to her, while for our other informants, Maria and Isabelle, there is no such ambiguity in the situation of the donors, so the unknown donor could be called father.

For a long time in Western societies, the genitors were the parents and the parents were the genitors. Sexuality, procreation, filiation and alliance coincided, as did the production and reproduction of the family. The father of the child was supposed to be the husband of the mother, the child of a married woman could pass for the child of her husband, whereas the child of an unmarried woman and a married man was a bastard. It was not nature (biology) that made this filiation, but marriage: the institution that provided the framework of procreation and of sexuality. Sexuality outside marriage was not permitted, which does not mean, of course, that it did not occur but that it had to be kept secret. We were in a filiative system within which the child's mother and the child's father were supposed to be its genitors and in which the making of a child and its reproduction overlapped, without, however, a clear delineation of the priority to be assigned to each of these two terms. Our conjuring trick, our symbolic construction, has been to make-believe that it is nature – the truth of the body – that created filiation, without recognising that it was the scaffolding of filiation and of the fabricating of the child within marriage that provided the validation. Yet, as family configurations have evolved, procreation could become separated from marriage and the making of children separated from the process of reproduction, even if the two elements are both essential for a child to reach adulthood. This is the same idea as that expressed by Boltanski when he wrote: 'only the confirmation by the spoken word confers on individuals a property that is essential for being recognised as human beings and which accounts for their uniqueness and which is their singularity' (Boltanski 2004: 71 (translation by Bolland)). When these two necessary conditions of filiation are not satisfied, what status is to be assigned to each of them? Can we still believe that the procreation of the child is the major reason for the child's filiation by still clinging to a conception of there being only two possible parents – a genitor father and a genitrix mother – whatever the alliance between them? Or can we conceive of children sometimes having four parents: a genitor and a father, a genitrix and a mother? Or, again, alongside parents to whom have devolved the role of parents and the parental functions, there could exist other figures required to come into the world, for example, the genitor/genitrix figures, who might perhaps be part of the child's biographical truth – for the child's body comes in part from them – yet without having any ties to the child's other parents. How should we designate them and distinguish between these two? Do we have to use the terms of reference mother and father for these genitor figures, who are not called upon to become parents on a daily basis, and reserve the terms of address Mummy and Daddy for the actual parents? For these latter parents also have the right to terms of reference.

It is not a matter of denying the biological – the gene, for example, clearly contains one kind of truth for people about their origins and personal identity. It is, rather, a matter of giving a place to the biological that reflects only the part it plays and which cannot and does not include the whole. Our parents do not originate in our genes. Human construction is not an object truth, even if knowing this object truth plays a part in the construction of the human being and his or her family identity. And, above all, I agree with Salazar's remark (this volume) that the virtue of genetic discourse is its capacity to bring people back to what they already know. For homosexual couples, what they know has nothing to do with scientific truth – actually the two parents cannot be the two genitors – and what they know they cannot use to make meaning in their society. However, they will use any other principle for family construction available to them – for instance, in Maria and Isabelle's situation, a cognatic system.

Notes

Translated by Patrick Bolland.
1. I choose to use 'homoparental families' and not 'homosexual families' to insist on the fact that it is not the family that is homosexual, but only the father or the mother.
2. Such as Weston (1991), Strathern (1992a), Gullestad and Segalen (1995), Ginsburg and Rapp (1995), Franklin and McKinnon (2001).
3. It is still difficult today to start any article on kinship without referring to Schneider: an example is in the book edited by Franklin and McKinnon (2001), in which the majority of the seventeen chapters focus, admittedly critically, on Schneider's *American Kinship* (Schneider, 1968).
4. For whom the question, 'Who is your father?' or 'Who is your mother?', which makes it possible to construct genealogies, does not have much meaning; or, at least, does not have the same meaning that we assign to it (see Meillassoux 2000).
5. Nor is Schneider concerned about the history behind this biological assertion. I am thinking here of Marcela Iacub's *L'Empire du ventre*, which is an attack on the increasing emphasis on childbirth to designate the true mother, to the detriment of the relationship by marriage, the legal relationship and non-biological ties (Iacub 2004).
6. See Mathieu (1991) for a collection of articles on this theme written between 1970 and 1989.
7. The text in French is: 'Là où manque la main de la parenté, qui rassemblait ceux qu'elle avait saisis, le mariage lance aussitôt son grappin pour ramener celui qui s'écarte.'
8. The text in French is : '[ce] sont ceux qui possèdent le secret des lieux et des temps, [ce] sont ceux qui ont prononcé les paroles requises ou accompli les gestes rituels, [ce] sont ceux encore que la vérité a choisis pour s'abattre sur eux: les prophètes, les devins, les innocents, les aveugles, les fous, les sages, etc.'.
9. In this case a family is 'constituted' with the arrival of the child and not 'reconstituted' some years later; and the child moving from one household to the other, between a female household and a male household, is a function of the prior agreement reached between the parents.
10. In France, adoption, while it is authorised for single people, is not permitted for unmarried couples: it is only granted to recognised, legal 'units'. At the same time, the donation of gametes, sperm or ova is not authorised for single people. As for access to surrogacy arrangements, this is illegal in France for all persons, regardless of their marital status. According to a survey

conducted by the Association des Parents et Futurs Parents Gays et Lesbiens (APGL 2001), of fifty children included in the survey born or adopted in a homosexual context, nearly half were the result of a co-parenting project; a third were born as a result of anonymous-donor artificial insemination, and slightly less than one-fifth through adoption.

11. I prefer the term 'unit' to that of 'a couple', unit being applicable to a single component – as in the case of single-parenting – or several elements composing a unit, while the term 'couple' reflects too narrowly a two-person unit.
12. Since 1997, I have been studying kinship with homosexual fathers and mothers. I have met about fifty couples. Isabelle, Maria and Amélie were amongst them. Of course, I have changed their names.
13. A man and a woman, usually a gay and a lesbian, each of them typically living with a partner, agree to have a child together and to be the legitimate father and mother, while still living in different households. This is a family configuration that approximates the reconstituted family, except that the family is together (constituted) from when the child is born.
14. The crèche is a public system of day care for very young children (from two months to three years, that is from between the end of maternity leave to admission to kindergarten). There are two types of crèche: those entirely run by early-childhood educators and the *crèches parentales*, in which a smaller group of early-childhood educators is supported by the children's parents, who take it in turn to be present with the children. In our case, it was a matter of Maria or Isabelle being present five hours a week as well as during meal times.
15. The law allowing parents to choose to give their child the name of the mother or the father, or the two names joined together by a double hyphen has only been effective since January 2005.
16. We should note that, on the one hand, the pacte de solidarité civile (civil solidarity pact or 'PaCS') had not yet been adopted when their children were born; on the other hand, this PaCS does not alter the civil status of the contracting parties or their heirs.
17. Except in assigning the child a ridiculous given name.
18. The legislation passed in March 2002: Article 377–1: 'The decision to confer delegation may foresee, for reason of the child-rearing of the child as for the mother and the father, or of one of these latter, that the two will share all or part of the exercise of parental authority with the delegated third party' (our translation). A third party can take on certain parental functions such as, for example, registering the child in a school (educational duties) or giving permission for the child to undertake a surgical intervention (ensuring the health of the child).
19. To summarise the French legal system of kinship we can say there are three ways to be in an alliance relationship: marriage, PaCS and cohabitation; and two ways to institute descent: descent by birth, with divisibility or not according to the alliance relationship, and descent by adoption, which can be plenary or simple. In addition to these ways of making kinship, we can add assisted reproductive technology.

Alliance relationship
(a) Marriage: this is only authorised for heterosexual people. It is a public act, celebrated in the town hall of one of the spouses, with ceremony, by the

mayor or his/her assistant. Since the date of marriage, the spouses form a unit for economic, social and symbolic things. Most of the time the wife takes her husband's surname, although this is not an obligation. To divorce, the spouses have to present themselves in front of a judge in a court tribunal in order to end their union and to separate the things they have held together. Generally, the wife cannot use her ex-husband's surname any more.

(b) PaCS ('Pacte de solidarité civil, civil partnership): this is a contract between two non-married people of the same or different sexes and was instituted in 1999. It is signed in a court tribunal without ceremony and establishes only economic and social solidarity between these two people.

(c) Consensual union or cohabitation: this is a common subsistence certificate between two non-married people, issued by the town hall in order for cohabitees to have some of the same economic advantages as married couples.

Descent

1. (a) Descent by birth for married people: a wife giving birth and becoming a mother transforms her husband into a father without any other declaration; this is called *'présoumption de paternité'* (presumed fatherhood). This kind of descent is qualified as *'filiation indivisible'*. Until 2005, the children had to take their father's surname, but, if their parents chose, they could use their mother's surname in daily life. However, since 2005, the parents can choose to give their children any one or both of their surnames. The parents share the parental authority and, even if they divorce, they usually jointly keep this authority.

(b) Descent by birth for a cohabitant mother and father: both of them have to declare they are the mother and the father of the child. Since 2005, this is no longer necessary for the mother: birth becomes descent. If the child's parents recognised their parenthood at the same time, the same rules apply as for married couple. If not, the child bears the name of the relative who recognised it first. The parents can also share parental authority.

2. Descent by adoption: this is recorded at a court tribunal.

(a) Descent by plenary adoption: this is only authorised by one entity, either a married couple or one person, whatever her/his sexuality; so this adoption is forbidden for homosexual or heterosexual cohabiting couples. This kind of adoption deletes the adopted child's birth parents. We can call it 'substitutive descent'. When a married couple adopt, the descent rules are the same as for descent by birth.

(b) Simple adoption: this is an additional descent – the birth parents are not deleted but lose their parental authority. The adopted child has to take the adopted parent's surname, but she/he can keep the first parent's surname as a second surname. This kind of adoption is useful when there is divorce and remarriage and if the parent in law wants to consider his/her child in law as an heir. Legally, simple adoption can be requested by married couples as well as 'PaCSed' or cohabitant couples, whatever their sexuality, but depends on the court tribunal judge.

Reconstituted families do not change the establishment of descent rules; the child can only have one mother and one father. But very recently (since 2002) parents in law can share parental authority with the first parents if they agree.

Assisted reproductive technology
The bioethics laws of 1994 authorise artificial insemination with the donation of sperm or oocyte – and now donation of the embryo – only to married couples or heterosexual cohabitants who have lived together for two years. The donor must remain anonymous. Surrogate motherhood is forbidden.

Looking at the French legal system of kinship, we can see that a single homosexual person can become a mother or father but not a homosexual couple.

20. The donor remains unknown to the mother, but his identity is known to the medical services, before the 1984 Bioethics Law, to gynaecologists and, following the adoption of this law, to the Centre de conservation du sperme (Cecos). Some psychologists of medically assisted reproductive services advise mothers to ask for the same sperm 'source' in order that the children become 'quasi-siblings', that is, stemming from the same donor.
21. Out of law, of course.
22. See Bestard (2004b) on the advantages of gamete-donor anonymity.

CHAPTER 6

CORPO-REAL IDENTITIES:
PERSPECTIVES FROM A GYPSY COMMUNITY

Nathalie Manrique

– You have to imagine, then, that there are two ruling powers, and that one of them is set over the intellectual world, the other over the visible … May I suppose that you have this distinction of the visible and intelligible fixed in your mind?

– I have. (Plato 1991: 250)

For a very long time, philosophers have been debating whether there is not one but two routes to reach truth: the empirical and the abstract. According to Bachelard (1993: 239 [1938]), 'we have to accept a real break between sensible knowledge and scientific knowledge' (my translation). For Bachelard, two categories of knowledge shape our understanding of the world. He called the first 'empirical knowledge' (*connaissance empirique*) and the second 'scientific knowledge' (*connaissance scientifique*). The understanding of truth, then, can take two different directions: on the one hand, 'rational interpretation [which] comes from the immediate observation of raw facts' (Héritier 1996: 150, my translation), 'facts of life' (Franklin 1997; Carsten 2001) or 'facts of nature' (Strathern 1992a) and, on the other hand, truth that emerges from abstraction. While 'empirical facts', according to Bachelard, are based on everyday life experiences, 'scientific facts' are built on scientific reality; that is, on a logical construction of the relationship between different observable facts by means of controlled experiments. The latter facts are immersed in a scientific language; a sort of metalanguage which, borrowing from Lévi-Strauss on myth, 'makes full use of discourse, but does so by situating its own significant oppositions at a higher level of complexity than that required by language operating for profane ends'

(1977: 66). Even if we do not conclude that scientific facts are similar to mythological narrative, as the former are based on experimental criteria which can be questioned and the latter need only faith to be considered true, these two discourses act at the same level. These metalanguages, by means of their systems of classification, place the symbolic order of humans and things at a level that can be separated from empirical facts and local representations of the world. That is why only specialists are supposed to know the rules or the 'significant oppositions' on which such knowledge is founded, in contrast with the 'facts of life', which can be verified by ordinary people.

This time-honoured philosophical discussion has interesting repercussions for the anthropology of kinship. Bodily identity is represented in Western societies through a merger of these two perceptions of truth, which are thus rendered indistinguishable: facts of life and scientific or mythological facts are merged in Western understandings of how an individual transmits identity to another and how the degree of proximity between two people is estimated.

Tools to Define Kinship: Blood and Genes

In Western societies, blood and genes are two concepts that symbolise kin relatedness and, consequently, corporeal identity. Indeed, to be related as kin is, above all, to share the 'same' (according to local and scientific representations of sameness) blood and/or genes. Moreover, blood and genes are the concepts on which Western notions of the reality of the ties between people are constructed.

However, the nature of these two concepts differs. Whereas blood is a bodily substance that everyone can see (a small cut on a finger can demonstrate its existence), genes are invisible for the majority of people.[1] Furthermore, blood, like breath, is indisputably a metaphor of life: to lose all one's blood means to die.[2] The genome, as it cannot be lost and is not directly observable, appears, then, to be less related to the working and living body. At first sight, knowledge of blood appears more obviously related to the 'facts of life' or the 'facts of nature' and to something more readily verifiable than genetics.[3] Genes appear to be more of an abstract construction created by experts initiated into certain ways of knowing and who attempt to understand the truth of biological transmission through particular tools. Indeed, since the beginning of the twentieth century, genes have become increasingly the essential instrument with which to provide irrefutable evidence of biological facts (see for example Franklin 2001: 306; Legrand 2004: 182–83).

But what are the procedures for transmitting blood or genetic identity? While the genetic material of each person is present in his or her gametes and male and female gametes only need to meet to make fertilisation possible, blood is not transmitted directly from the male to the female body. Blood is not, as such, a factor in conception. There are societies, however, where blood identity is thought to be inherited from parents and where 'relatedness by blood' is significant. In these cases, the seed, more often than not the sperm, is semantically linked to blood.[4] Such a representation of biological transmission is closely related to local representations of the wider social world, which includes values and perceptions of how identity is transmitted. To put it in a nutshell, we can say that non-expert understandings of the world play on two levels. First, they are based on what are considered to be 'raw facts', which everybody should be able to observe (and here truth is based on what is thought to be shared experiences of life). Secondly, these empirical facts are immersed in local values, which are generally different from scientific values. The latter come about as a result of experimentation carried out by specialists and appear to be closer to the 'rational' truth than to 'empirical facts', which in turn become 'irrational' (according to Bachelard's definition of rationality). In the context of transmitting identity, public understandings of blood and genes are enmeshed in this dichotomy but they spill over from one category to another. Indeed, as we have seen, blood is observably a bodily substance and its obvious link to life gives it a vital attribute which readily comes to symbolise the transmission of life. Genes appear to be further away than blood from the 'facts of life', even though they 'naturally' transmit identity, which makes the idea of genetic inheritance a less obvious social construction than the transmission of blood.

The way in which identity is transmitted is intrinsically related to both empirical or biological facts and the local metalanguage. This enables some people, dealing with empirical and/or scientific criteria, to construct their own truth based on their representation of scientific knowledge combined with local ideas.[5] According to Dorfles (1975: 198–99), '[w]e have to accept, in the final analysis, the hypothesis that there is diversity in man's state of consciousness, perception, ideation and imagination, depending on the period and the cultures in which he is situated' (my translation). This diversity also exists within the same period and within the same culture as well as in the same individual, depending on the socio-psychological context in which he or she is situated (Elster 1977). It is no wonder, then, that representations of proximity between kin are also diverse.

Let me introduce a debate that took place in Spain during my fieldwork.[6] A couple claimed the right to challenge what Hermida and Pereiro (1997) call the 'most ancestral taboo of humanity' by living together in the name of love despite the fact that they were brother and sister.[7] They said that they found out they were siblings after they had fallen in love, and then they were unable to live apart from one another. When the woman became pregnant, they were both afraid she would give birth to an 'abnormal' child. Therefore, they decided to have genetic tests carried out on the embryo. Doctors diagnosed the fetus as 'normal' and the couple decided to keep the child and not to have an abortion. Furthermore, from then onwards they stopped hiding their relationship and decided to live like a 'real family' and to have their relationship publicly recognised by claiming a civil marriage: it was as if for them the genetic tests were the proof that, despite the vigorous public debate their situation had provoked and which continues today (a film is now being made of their lives (see Ortiz 2005)), the relationship was not after all so bad. Moreover, it could not be considered bad for it was based on love: 'We fell in love and for us it was the most important thing' (Fourmont 2003, my translation). Indeed, they pointed out that they would not have fallen in love if they had known they were siblings, thus drawing on the commonly shared idea in Western societies that the idea of incest repels (Westermarck 1901; Roscoe 1994). Their first child, who at the time of the report was a young teenage girl and who had a younger brother, also responded to the notion of incest in a Westermarckian manner: 'That could not happen to us. It is completely different because my brother and I have been brought up together. It could happen if, as was the case with our parents, we had not been brought up together' (Fourmont 2003, my translation). Genetic tests showed that people can practise incest and still claim social legitimacy: the couple were above all parents of a 'normal' child. Unexpectedly, the juxtaposition of several facts considered to be true because they belong to 'the facts of nature' (to feel revolted by incest and that incest produces malformations) turns genetics into proof that the common understanding of incest is false and that sexual relations between siblings can be considered 'normal'. It can also demonstrate that genetic propinquity is not enough to define closeness. Public understanding of science, by giving an empirical interpretation of scientific facts (the birth of a 'genetically normal' child), becomes a tool used against scientific assertions concerning kinship closeness. In this way, to be associated with truth, genetics has to be verified empirically and vice versa. People can then clearly create their own frameworks for understanding how identity is transmitted.

Gypsy Corpo-real Identity

To develop the points introduced above, I move to a Gypsy community in Morote and San Juan, Spain. Morote (which has nearly 9,000 inhabitants, of whom approximately 800 are Gypsies) and San Juan (which has nearly 4,600 inhabitants, including approximately 450 Gypsies) are located in the south of Spain, near Granada. In the past, Gypsies from these small towns practised trades mainly connected with horses, donkeys and mules. Today, this particular population, like the majority of Spanish Gypsies, is sedentary even if their economic activity as farm labourers obliges them to travel frequently.

I once asked Felicita, a fifty-five-year-old Gypsy woman, about the influence of the father's and the mother's contribution to creating a child. She was taken aback by my question and answered: 'You must know that the two parents both contribute to making the child. The proof lies in the fact that you can analyse blood to find out who is the father and the mother of any child. You also know that the doctors can say who the parents are.' For Felicita, something that can be found in the blood makes the relationship between a child and his or her parents indisputable. This 'something' reveals genealogical ties and the transmission of identity. For her, the proof of this is that doctors, people who have this kind of knowledge, can find such links by analysing blood. And I, as a 'teacher', so as a 'quasi-scientist', should know that.[8] Here, the discourse of blood, like genetics, works as a metalanguage.

Local representations of procreation involving the blending of men's and women's blood (semen and menses) in the female belly are congruent with Felicita's perceptions. She appears to raise the evidence of paternity and maternity based on blood to the same level as genetic knowledge. In this sense, Gypsy representations of how identity is transmitted are not contrary to representations of genetic inheritance. Sometimes, in the imprecision of the concept of kinship in Western societies (ties can be constructed on a variety of things such as blood, breeding and shared names), the use of blood metaphors can have unexpected consequences. For the Gypsies of Morote and San Juan, the similarity or difference carried in the blood is the essential marker that defines how close one person is to another. But the metaphor of blood, like some idioms of flesh (see Porqueres i Gené and Wilgaux, this volume), can also be used in a way which implies that bodily identity is not only linked to one's genealogy but also to one's affinity. Indeed, even if blood ties are essential in defining identity in the Gypsy community, to be a mother is not only to be related through blood to one's offspring but also to be both a wife (that is, as we shall see, to be 'blood-fed' by legitimate sexual relations) and able to feed a child (hence the importance of the role of nurturing and breeding to complete 'consanguine' ties).[9] Blood is the vehicle of filial and affinal closeness. This similarity does not mean that a wife and a husband become biologically identical (of the same blood) or that they create kinship ties with each other and become genetically the same. I note here, as both Edwards (2000) and Bestard (this volume) have, that blood sameness like biological sameness, is not always synonymous with genetic sameness: the notion of blood carries more symbolic significance than that of genes. In the Gypsy case, it is not only related to filiation but also to affinity: to transmit blood is to nurture someone else during sexual intercourse, and to create filial and affinal ties. Sexual acts are thought to be not only about procreation but also about nurturing relations.

A study of Gypsy ways of representing the transmission of blood reveals a tension between empirical knowledge, which demonstrates the identical role of men and women in conception (in their contribution of blood), and mythological knowledge, which, by highlighting male supremacy in procreation, appears to be intrinsically tied to ideology. The idea of male dominance in procreation emerges in how masculinity is seen to be dynamic and femininity inert. The perception of dynamism and inertia is also embedded in the act of giving, where the giver is thought to act on the receiver's body (as in sexual relations, where a man acts on the woman's body by giving his procreative substance).

Inertia and Dynamism

For the Gypsies of Morote and San Juan, dynamism is highly valued and is strongly emphasised. It is foundational to Gypsy social hierarchy. Although men are supposed to be 'naturally' active (as seen by the outpouring of semen) and women less active, it is not rare to hear women expressing pride in the effort they put into carrying out certain activities. Indeed, activity in general is strongly valued. Thus, good workers are admired by all and are regarded as being worthy of confidence and meriting interest.

During a conversation between neighbours, Rubén, a small eleven-year-old boy who wished to present a positive image of his maternal grandfather, insisted on his incredible capacity for work in spite of having had one of his legs amputated. Alicia, an eighteen-year-old girl, fulminated against her friend Piedad who was disconcerted. It turned out that Piedad's brother, a Gypsy from Asturias (in the north of Spain), had written a letter to Alicia in which he declared his passion for her and described how he wanted to find a well-paying job in order to prevent her from working. She protested: 'Who does he think he is? I want to work. I will not remain idle while he's working.'

The perception of female dynamism is not necessarily shared by all Spanish Gypsies. In San Juan and Morote, women are required to demonstrate their activity, while men are often defined by their active character and are not required to justify what they are (see Lagunas Arias (2000) for the case of Gypsies from Catalonia). This male quality confers on them an active role in procreation. Felicita explained: 'The father makes the child and the mother places herself so that he will do this to her'. The sexual act is considered above all the dynamic relation, with the man acting on the woman's body. An energetic copulatory movement is considered to be of primary importance for procreation. Thus, jokingly, one woman told me that one of her *consuegras* (her son's mother-in-law), at the time fifty-five years old and thus certainly menopausal, 'became pregnant because she made love very vigorously'. This joke shows the importance of vigorous movement, which in this case made pregnancy possible without the menses even though, according to Gypsy understandings, the menses are essential for conception. Gypsy women point out that this is the reason children look more like their father than their mother.

Nevertheless, and somewhat paradoxically, men attribute a particular generative-reproductive force to women. They say that newborn children resemble their mothers more than their fathers. Thus, men generally allege that the child of a Gypsy father and a non-Gypsy mother will resemble a *Payo* (a non-Gypsy) and that a child of a *Payo* father and a Gypsy mother will resemble a Gypsy.[10] Yet men consider themselves to have an active influence on the physical appearance of their offspring. Indeed, according to them, the greater the intensity of the 'blows (*golpes*)' a man makes in the vagina, the greater the extent to which the child will resemble him. To make love like *Payos*, for example, that is, with less intensity, will produce taller children with light skin who look like *Payos*. The vigorousness of male sexual activity modifies the 'natural' properties of resemblance of the female substance. This gender distinction is based on the greater or lesser importance given to the active role of each of them in conception and not on the fact that they are referring to men or women, even if men generally consider that women make a more significant contribution to procreation since it is they who give birth.[11] Joseío, an eighty-year-old man, after having told me that children look like their mothers, explained that, after all, in a 'crossed' marriage, the children always resemble Gypsy since the Gypsy blood is stronger (more active) than the *Payo*.

Women, in contrast, mainly stress the active power of male fertilisation. For them, a child more closely resembles the individual who has provided most of the work at the time of conception (despite the fact that semen and menses contribute to the fetal matter). This discourse, only superficially contradictory, that is, in the form used to express the distinction but not in its consequences, is often ignored by the opposite sex. Thus, without intending to, on three occasions I caused conflict between a married couple when, after arriving at the point of asking the woman about conception, the husband, hearing his wife's answer, picked a quarrel with her by maintaining the opposite. Similarly, women do not envisage that they contribute more than their husband to the appearance of their child.

The different views on how appearance is transmitted, linked to who is the more dynamic partner in procreation, reveal the fact that empirical knowledge differs according to context (in this case according to the gender of the speaker), but that context does not influence mythological facts: dynamism determines which individual has the dominant role in procreation.

Fruitful Bleedings

For the Gypsies of Morote and San Juan, identity, mainly transmitted through dynamism in sexual intercourse, is carried in the blood. In order to procreate, sperm and menstrual blood have to coalesce inside the belly of a woman who has periods. Indeed, for Gypsies, sexual intercourse between a man and a woman during her menses is essential for a 'normal' conception, even if women recount stories of parthenogenesis. Joaquina, for example, told me that to procreate: 'It must be during your menstruation.' Then, at that moment, through the influence of the sperm, the menses coagulate to create the fetus, which Gypsies consider to be like an already-formed child in miniature.

In fact, the male principle, which is considered to be like a divine principle (comparable to the descriptions by Delaney (1991) and Fortier (2001) in two Muslim societies), is seen as providing life. After talking about the agency of her husband's semen in the coagulation process, Esperanza added that subsequently 'God coagulates it all (*todo lo cuaja el Señor*)'. Similarly, when speaking about the creation of the first Gypsy, a man during our conversation suddenly used the terms 'the Gypsy (*el Gitano*)' referring to God, thereby making an analogy between Gypsy men and God. He presented the parallel between the seminal fluid and the divine principle spontaneously, thus conferring a supernatural character to the male substance. One of the properties of semen, then, is to give life and the menses need to be fertilised for procreation to occur.

After conception takes place, the semen becomes the vehicle of life, which spreads gradually through the woman's belly. Antonio said: 'The more you put in, the more it [the fetus] becomes alive.' Esperanza, his wife, clarified: 'The husband has to do it [to give life] little by little until he has finished, like a machine.' In fact, it appears that the fetus becomes alive immediately, once coagulation has occurred, but that life has to develop progressively thanks to the dynamic and repeated introduction of semen into the maternal body – Gypsies speak about 'work' in this context. For Gypsies, procreation is spontaneous but life, like everything else in the world, needs progressive growth through feeding, that is, through work. Josefa explained that the fetus is completely alive when it is four or five months old, when it starts to move around in the belly, and that this is the result of the father's 'work' on the mother's body.

The vital contribution also takes place at the time of non-procreative sexual relations but then it is like feeding, providing nourishment for the female body and not the fetus. Semen is seen as a vital reproductive substance, which by means of mechanistic movement fertilises and nourishes the woman's body during her period of fertility, which is when sexual relations are truly legitimate. Thus, women make fun of women who perform what they call their 'marital duty': they say that their weight increases and their buttocks get chubby. It is interesting here to draw a parallel with Gypsy representations of health, youth and beauty, which are expressed in the same terms. When a woman becomes pregnant, women say 'she has her belly full', but this expression is also used to refer to a woman who has just had sexual intercourse. In fact, women who are said to grow bigger after sex are those who cannot give birth (infertile women) or who cannot bear any more children (following the menopause). Unused semen is thought to be stored in women's bodies, making them grow bigger and rejuvenating them. 'She has become so young! (*que nueva se ha puesto*).' In addition, women recognise men who have frequent sexual intercourse by their thinness. The male vital substance is a limited quantity, for which men have to compensate by consuming certain foods that are known to increase the quantity of blood.

The Seed of Wind

Semen is conceptualised as a gas or breath. Indeed, according to the Gypsies of San Juan and Morote, it comes from the lungs (whereas menses originate in the woman's belly). This relation between air and seminal fluid appears all the more clearly in Gypsy vocabulary where the word *ril* is used to designate bodily wind and the verb *rilar*, which is the verbal form of the same root, to refer to sexual relations. The movements of the fetus (the fruit of the sexual act) are also thought to be similar to those of a bloated belly. Most Gypsies only talk about 'that (*eso*)' in a whisper or use the word *sangre* (blood) to designate the seminal fluid. Some prefer the term *leche* (milk), which is used by the local non-Gypsy population. One woman designated it by the words *gasoleo* and *gasolina* (petrol), perhaps because of the derivation from 'gas'. But they do not usually adopt a specific term to designate the man's seed, even if its gaseous quality emerges clearly in their discourses (and they do not use the conventional Spanish term, as they do for menses).

In addition, Gypsy men in San Juan and Morote say with a smile that, according to Gypsies in the past, their earliest ancestors emerged from a kick that God gave to a *cajonera* (horse shit) and, as he did this, God broke wind.[12] The association between the gaseous principle and fertilisation is explicit here. Caterina Pasqualino (1998) found a parallel between semen and the breath of Flamenco singers, who are usually men. It is said that their breath has the capacity of fertilisation by descending into women's entrails.

Furthermore, as semen (the men's 'blood') is perceived as nutriment, Gypsies seek to increase their blood by swallowing foods that have the ability to control the quantity of gas present in their body. On the one hand, they enjoy certain foods which they consider to have the capacity to inflate the belly (such as chickpeas, potatoes and rotting meat). On the other hand, they use certain carminative plants (such as fennel, basil and mint) by which they can control gas excesses and avoid gas expulsions and thus are able to retain their semen – the vital nutriment – inside the body.[13] This particular perception of semen, and similarly with the menses, is linked to the local hierarchy between men and women in Gypsy society (see also Delaney 1991).

Wasted Blood?

Women's blood also takes part in procreation through menses. Menses, however, do not nourish the bodies of men. Semen and menstrual blood are nevertheless likened in a natural way and both are referred to by the same words *sangre* and *reglas* (menses): in the case of semen, an analogy is made with the bleeding of women. The perception of the coalescence of two bloods is founded on the empirical observation of two types of outpourings: the male (semen) and the female (menses).

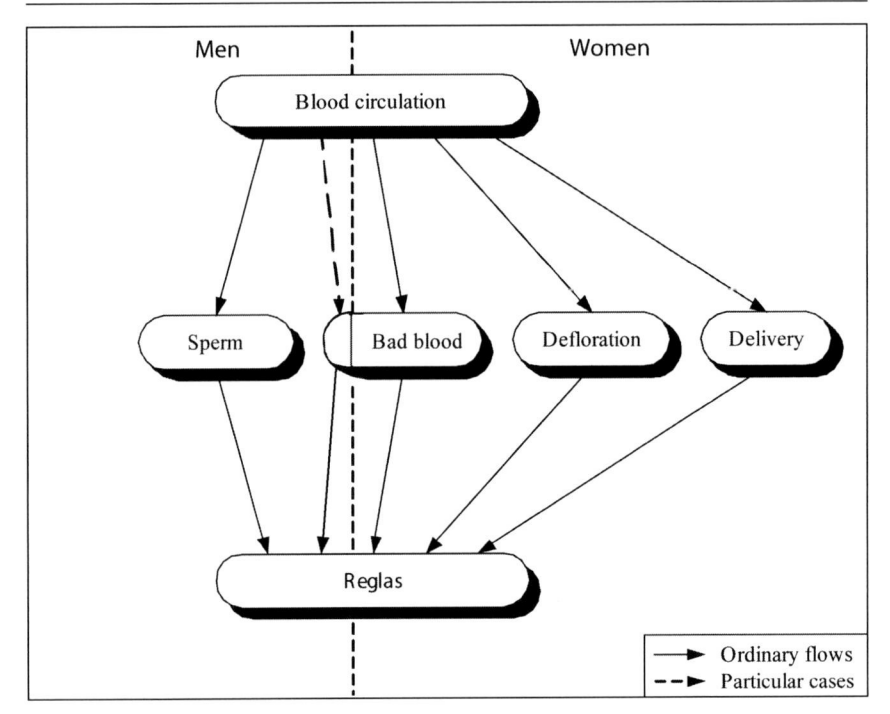

Figure 6.1. Blood flows

Only menses, however, produce 'bad blood (*sangre mala*)' (Fig. 6.1.), which is a residue of the women's circulatory blood. Indeed, contrary to men, women require a periodic purification. The arrow for the *sangre mala* resulting from the circulatory blood of men refers only to haemophiliacs, who purge incest or other transgressions of their parents by bleeding, and this is sanctioned by God.

It is not thought that men, who have no menses, are able to renew their blood, which, in any event, does not need renewing. In spite of the perception of menstrual blood as bodily waste, it is the symbol of women's fertility and for that reason the menarche is an important stage in the lives of Gypsy women. The first appearance of a girl's period is a matter of joy within the close family and provokes the observation, 'She is now a woman (*Ya es una mujer*).' The menarche puts her in the category of marriageable girls, which in this community is considered to be a very positive status (except by the girls' mothers, who always consider their daughter to be too young to leave home).[14]

It is perceived that women can only conceive at the time of their menses and this consequently gives this kind of blood a fertilising quality. It puts it on a similar level to semen. Indeed, fertilisation only takes place at the time of a double humoral flow. Semen and menstrual blood are perceived as two seeds (contrary to Aristotle (1979)) that need movement to coalesce. Moreover, the pregnant woman does not need to be purged any more. Her residual blood mixes with her husband's semen and benefits from its positive generative value. A pregnant woman does not produce 'bad blood' any longer because she is making the child. At this point, the blood flow is given a bodily explanation that is compatible with its function in reproduction (it is 'bad blood' only when it does not achieve its task of procreation (and see Douglas 1970: 53)).

Other forms of women's blood are also perceived as essential flows directly related to the different stages of reproduction. Hence blood coming from defloration and the blood released during childbirth have a bodily function associated with the cycle of procreation and for this reason are also not 'bad bloods'. The blood of menopausal women no longer flows from their bodies, so they can no longer procreate and sexual intercourse is therefore considered to be no longer essential. Nevertheless, menopausal and post-menopausal women are often accused of not being able to control their overflow of desire, as if they become more masculine at this stage of their life. One of the most common insults is to declare for all to hear that a particular older woman has put on weight, which suggests that she continues to 'sleep' with her husband.

Several men with whom I spoke proudly revealed that they took part in the birth of all their children, sometimes by cutting the umbilical cord. The blood of childbirth does not appear to repel Gypsy men in any way. The blood of childbirth is 'in its place' in Gypsy constructions of appropriate procreation. The fact that women's periods are considered to be 'bad blood' confirms the intrinsic association between being a woman, a wife and a genitrix and, consequently, women's place as the receptacle of both substance and movement, which places them in a lower position in the symbolic order. The hierarchical scale based on the predominance of each blood in procreation is also used to classify different degrees of proximity in terms of identity and to differentiate between Gypsy and non-Gypsy populations.

Blood Propinquity

As the fertile substances of men and women are of the same nature and origin, their mixing in the belly cannot be independent from Gypsy representations of identical and different bodies.[15] In fact, independent from the transmission of resemblance, Gypsies consider that the bonds of proximity depend on the degree to which the same blood is shared (Gay y Blasco 1999). Bloods need to be neither very close nor too distant in order to coagulate well. Thus a marriage between a Gypsy and a *Payo*, with either the man or the woman a Gypsy, would result in a child who is 'different'. In this connection, Esperanza told me that, when older Gypsies talked about a boisterous child who was 'mixed (*mezclado*)', or 'crossed (*cruzado*)', they said: 'Don't you see that he has the tail of a *Payo* (*no ve que tiene rabo de Payo*)?' Joseío also told me that the mixture of different bloods is not beneficial and gave the example of the mule, which is a product of a mare and a donkey and is generally sterile. The mixture of blood which provides life can only take place 'normally' between Gypsies. Mari Luz explained that the difference between a Gypsy and a *Payo* 'is carried in the blood (*se lleva en la sangre*)'. Difference in ethnicity is based on a greater difference between blood and consequently on a greater distance from close kin. Marriages between 'blood' relations make it possible to preserve one's Gypsy identity, and being of the same blood is to belong to the same genealogical network, which extends as far as first cousins.

However, unions that are too close are to be avoided. Tionila, a Gypsy woman who is about sixty years old, told me: 'Blood cannot be formed because it is already made.' This means that sexual relations create similarity in blood which can then coagulate. If this similarity pre-exists, that is, if two bloods are already the same, they cannot coagulate. Only when sexual partners are not of identical blood can they procreate. Female blood is transformed so that it becomes more similar to the male blood but it is not identical,[16] otherwise sexual relations would be incestuous – neither blood that is too different nor blood that is too identical can result in a 'good' coagulation.

To summarise, the transmission of identity rests to a greater or lesser degree in sharing the same blood. This is the principle of 'truthfulness' in defining Gypsy relatedness and is revealed in marriage prohibitions, incest and mixed marriages.

Fertilisation and Procreation: the Blending of Empirical and Mythological Facts

Even if the male contribution to procreation is enhanced by men's physical role in sexual intercourse, the contribution of the woman is not completely ignored. Women commonly say that at the time menstruation occurs sexual desire is stimulated. They consider this to be proof that they are more fertile during menstruation.[17] As I have argued, sexual desire is generally considered to be a male attribute (see Gay y Blasco 1999; Lagunas Arias 2000). Indeed the very feminine property of menstruation (menses represents the passage from childhood to womanhood) allocates to women a more active status than their 'normal' passive status. Women can procreate during menstruation and, since male qualities are essentially active, women are considered to be fertile when they have desire, that is, when they are active like men.

In considering Gypsy attachment to empirical knowledge, I put forward the hypothesis that when women's blood becomes most manifestly active (during menstruation) they are entering into their active 'male' phase. As menses come from the circulatory blood made from both father's and mother's genetic substance, and as periods are seen, like semen, to be an outpouring of blood, it is as if the menstrual flow has the capacity to activate the blood (semen) of the woman's father and her maternal grandfather. This explains why women can conceive only during menstruation and it also explains why Joseío can maintain that the offspring of a Gyspy woman and a *Payo* is a Gyspy child. The male, active property of the Gypsy woman's blood during her menstruation is, according to Joseío, stronger than the *Payo* blood. Procreation is therefore empirically and ideologically predominantly a masculine affair – the consequence of the mixing of two active/masculine bloods – even if it is through the woman's body.

This kind of fertility can be so powerful that women think that in some special circumstances they can become pregnant without the contribution of men. 'Sexlessness' (not having sexual relations) and fertilisation (coagulation) thus become two concepts that can coincide. Indeed, a certain form of parthenogenesis is possible where it is not semen that produces the coagulation of the menses in the belly of a woman (married or single). I was told stories by Gypsy women who had heard about other Gypsy women who had become pregnant without sexual intercourse (Manrique 2004). They described how one Gypsy woman in San Juan who was having her period got a fright when a snake passed between her legs as she walked to work in the tall grass. She said that people who were near her at that moment might have laughed and said to her that now she had her 'belly full (*la panza llena*)', in other words, that she was pregnant. The sight of a snake and the dread it conveyed could have coagulated the menses and produced a 'creepy-crawly (*un bicho*)' instead of a fetus inside the woman's stomach. Likewise, if a menstruating woman while kneading bread or dough moves her belly towards the edge of the table in a movement similar to that of sexual intercourse it could also result in conception. A woman can become 'full' with a *bicho* from such things. Note that it is not children who are born from parthenogenesis, but *bichos* which will be born lifeless or die in a short time. Indeed, through dynamism but without the contribution of the vital male substance which only men can provide, these conceptions can simulate fertilisation but cannot create a child. This singular kind of fertilisation highlights the important capacity of women to conceive but not to procreate. To procreate women need a masculine contribution, which has to be external to their body. Gypsy understandings of conception demonstrate, on the one hand, the possibility that women can be fertilised independently (they do not need a man to coagulate their blood) and, on the other hand, that women need real sexual intercourse to procreate (to give life to a child and not to a *bicho*). To be real mothers as opposed to only 'genetrixes' women need marriage (see Cadoret 2000). While women can fertilise (or be fertilised), they cannot create filiation: they cannot procreate by themselves. Here, then, the 'genetrix' is distinguished from the mother: she can conceive but she cannot have children.

The process of fertilisation does not necessarily give a woman the rights or duties to nurture a child; only legitimate sexual relations can do that. A discontinuity emerges between each of these roles in procreation. The dualism of fertilisation and procreation is fragmented, and the male part of women's menstrual blood is not strong enough to procreate – it does not carry life and human properties like 'pure' semen. Only marriage can allow a woman to acquire her reproductive integrity – to be a mother and to nurture a child. Men, in contrast, can reproduce without women, or so it is told in the myth in which the first Gypsy is the fruit of a man. Men possess an integrated procreative quality – they fertilise and procreate through the same movement and, for them, there is no disjuncture between fertilisation and procreation. As Degnen (this volume) writes, '[b]oth "food" and "body" already hold, carry and reproduce meaning about society and culture as well as significant roles in the symbolic world that humans use to demarcate social difference and similarity in everyday social life'. The Gypsy case, where marriage and procreation for a woman mean that she is nourished by a man, makes the roles of men and women in the transmission of identity (and of kinship) clear.

Since women, like men, possess generative matter they can also acquire masculine qualities. The use of the same word, *reglas*, for menses and semen demonstrates that we cannot conclude that there is a biological distinction between men and women but rather there is a discriminatory social representation of the place each occupies in social organisation and in the means to procreate (Héritier 1996). As Demény (this volume) demonstrates: 'Differentiations of social identities are also connected with the exercise of power.'

Despite the empirical knowledge about two kinds of outpourings that are the basis for the transmission of identity, it is ideological knowledge that underlines men's role in the perpetuation of human beings. Thus rules of marriage are founded on an empirical vision of two blood transmissions, whereas social organisation and the ideological classification of the world (dynamism and inertia; to nourish and to be nourished) on which it depends are androcentric. But, as we have seen, there is no contradiction between empirical knowledge and ideology: the two outpourings of blood can be considered to be masculine.

Gypsy representations of how identity is transmitted are meaningful in the process of how social positions (for example, a hierarchy between men and women) and boundaries between close and less close people (to be inside or outside kinship, for example) are constructed. For Gypsies of Morote and San Juan, kinship sameness is based on corpo-real truth, that is, on the sharing of a particular bodily element (blood), which, like genes in the case of the couple of siblings that we have considered before, is considered to be a verifiable fact, by either empirical or scientific tools.

Notes

I am very grateful to Patrick Bolland for his revision of my English in a previous version of this chapter and to Jeanette Edwards, Carles Salazar, Enric Porqueres i Gené and Auksuole Čepaitienė for their very fruitful comments.

1. As Janet Carsten (2001: 37) explains, the English word 'substance' is polysemic: 'Substance ... can denote a separate thing (that is, a person or body part); a vital part or essence of that thing or person; and also corporeal matter more generally, the tissue or fluid of which bodies are embodied.' The ambiguity of this term will allow me to play on two of the different senses of the notion of blood in the

context of Gypsy representations of the body – as both 'vital part' and 'corporeal matter'.
2. In some societies, such as the Gyspies of Morote and San Juan, the circulation of blood and breath are symbolically equivalent.
3. In the case of assisted conception, Marre and Bestard (this volume) point out that resemblance can be used by ordinary people as a tool to verify genetic truth.
4. This is generally the case in European societies, such as Lithuania (Čepaitienė, this volume), Norway (Melhuus and Howell, this volume), England (Edwards 2000) and Spanish Gypsies (Manrique 2004). This also seems to be the case in North America (Schneider 1968; Ragoné 1999) and in central Africa (Héritier 1996).
5. Compare how motherhood is represented by the foster-mothers studied by Demény (this volume).
6. I stayed for two years in Morote, between 1996 and 1998, and almost four months in San Juan, in 2000.
7. See also Xanthakou (2000) and Zonabend (2000) for ways in which incest between siblings is represented in Greece and in the north of France.
8. I explained to them that I was studying their culture, and, as I was too old to be a pupil, they chose to consider me as a teacher: *la maestra* became one of my nicknames.
9. This is similar to Godelier's (1982) analysis of Baruya's representation of sexuality even if, for the Gypsies, seminal nourishment does not imply fellatio.
10. I choose to use the Gypsy term to qualify non-Gypsy people and the non-Gypsy term to designate Gypsies. As Poutignat and Streiff-Fenart (1995) explain, the 'ethnic' term is always used to designate people who are different from oneself. This is the case in these two towns where Gypsies and non-Gypsies have no terms of their own to qualify themselves.
11. See Edwards (2004) for the perceived 'naturalness of gestation and birth' in England.
12. At first I thought that this story was a joke, but several Gypsy men told me the same story. Back in Paris, I read in Courthiade (2004) that very similar stories are told amongst Carpathian Gypsy groups.
13. They also use cardoon and poppy buds (the milk secretions of the first have the property of coagulating milk). We also know that in Europe the manufacture of cheese was associated with the conception of a child (Aristotle 1979; Belmont 1988). The relationship between poppy buds and blood is made through their shared colour.
14. See also Gamella (1996) for his general study of Andalusian Gypsies.
15. See in particular Françoise Héritier (1994).
16. Indeed, it is probable that Gypsies consider that a woman's blood becomes progressively the same as her husband's. That could explain why only the eldest child has these particular relationships with his/her maternal family and why a widow can transmit the surname of her husband's family: usually after the death of the man who carries the surname, it is forbidden for relatives to use the surname.
17. This perception of conception, fundamentally linked to menstrual flow, is quite uncommon, and all the more so in the discourse of Gypsy populations where, according to many anthropological studies, men reject female blood – that is, where women are required to avoid men when they are menstruating or have just given birth (see, for example, Williams 1981; and Okely 1983 on English Traveller Gypsies).

CHAPTER 7

INCEST, EMBODIMENT, GENES AND KINSHIP

Enric Porqueres i Gené and Jérôme Wilgaux

> The thing that'd worry me more [pause] is the chances of a natural brother and sister meeting [pause]. You know, a lot of these laboratories producing sperm might not be ethical. (Cited in Edwards 2004: 767)

The main aim of this chapter is to explore the heuristic implications of ideas about shared substances in an analysis of the 'new genetics'. While looking at the continuities and discontinuities created by genetic, and particularly 'new genetic', paradigms, we examine some of the current thinking on the status of individuality and the person by analysing the prohibition of incest which has been central to various traditions in the anthropology of kinship. In so doing, this chapter addresses two interrelated criticisms of current anthropological kinship theory: first, that new forms of *relatedness* represent a radical break from 'traditional kinship' and, secondly that Western cultural understandings of kinship are radically different from non-Western *ones*.

Modernity and Kinship Relationships

At the beginning of the 1990s, a number of influential researchers, such as Marilyn Strathern (1992a, b) and Sarah Franklin (1997, 2001), put forward the idea that we are in a sort of 'post period', which we read to mean a period marked by a radical rupture with the past. From this perspective, the Western past (as well as non-Western systems of kinship) is characterised by the centrality of kin relatedness in contrast to the contemporary Western world, which is marked by the centrality of the individual – at the expense of kinship. We believe that this contrast is inaccurate, although it is clear that the contemporary context is characterised by new possibilities for establishing kinship, with an increase in, amongst other things, international adoption and ways in which gay men and lesbians can create families, both of which illustrate how individual choice is reinforced and the notion of individual agency strengthened. Nevertheless, we disagree with the idea that the present-day situation frames qualitatively new categories of relationships, resulting in an epistemological break with the past.

With the publication of David Schneider's *American Kinship* in 1968, an old and often-repeated anthropological representation of contemporary Western patterns of kinship was reinforced: namely the consideration that Western culture is fundamentally different from the rest of human cultural experience. The same theme appeared in Strathern's *After Nature* (1992a), where contemporary English culture is depicted as a process of increasing separation between fields previously embedded. Strathern identifies a process of 'literalisation', which is deeply inscribed in Western middle-class culture and which supposes that by clearing away assumptions the truth can be reached. Strathern also argues that the person is normally not defined by kinship alone. Other kinds of social relations and choice are central to her analysis of relatedness in both the English and Melanesian contexts she addresses. For Strathern, the contemporary rupture stems from a radical autonomisation of the *individual* that comes from an over-focalisation on the body. In an important paper, where she forgets to mention the eventual effects of adoption in current conceptions on Western kinship, Strathern restates her main point about the very contemporary irreversible processes set off by uncovering traditional assumptions: 'while the procreative act is constitutive of kinship in a biogenetic sense, making that knowledge explicit makes more not less evident the fact that the social relationship is contingent. What once underpinned Euro-American understandings of kinship now alters the place that social relationships held in ideas about primordial personal identity' (1995: 360).

This point is clearly made in her analysis of the new techniques of visualisation applied to embryos. The embryo emerges as a kind of precocious *sujet de droit* – a legally recognized entity – independent of his or her social relations. The same point was made by Franklin (1993) in her analysis of the debates surrounding the British 'Human Fertilisation and Embryology Act' introduced in 1989 and enacted in 1990. Here she shows how the embedded fields of genealogy and the pragmatics of social distinction that are specific to traditional English kinship are replaced by the legitimacy of only biological truth, which results from the cognitive separation of biological facts. As a result, the individual emerges as a natural and unique combination of genetic information, stemming from other unique individuals. In this way, the idea of a constitutive relationship fades and is replaced by the absolute affirmation of embodied individuality, which is thought to be present from the beginning of life and which, in turn, carries value and merits juridical respect. The embryo (actually the pre-embryo) is deemed to be an individual from the beginning and is presented as an uncontested fact, while relations between individuals, even parent-children relations, are increasingly subject to discussion and thereby increasingly questionable. Debates on the biogenetic truth of filiation in the context of adoption or medically assisted reproduction are particularly eloquent, with the offspring emerging as an undeniable *sujet de droit*, whereas relations between individuals appear to be essentially conventional. Hence, while the dignity of the embryo or the adopted child is a given, the right to establish filiation links is submitted to discussion and regulation. In this way relations are thus being built after the natural facts and are located 'after nature'.[1]

We agree with these authors in considering that such images and representations pose important problems for cultural continuity. This is particularly clear in the obstacles being raised against the right to abortion, deriving partly from the undermining of the earlier idea that, up to some advanced point in pregnancy, the fetus is a part of the mother's body. There is no doubt that we are confronted with new and common representations that shape our cognitive and emotional maps of the social world. But scholars such as Strathern and Franklin, while succeeding in identifying important trends in contemporary ways of understanding the rights of the embryo, in our opinion go too far. We argue that they are in fact proposing a doubly fallacious account: one concerning changes over time in Western kinship and the other concerning the crisis in anthropological kinship theory.

On the one hand, the supposed radical novelty of the emergence of the rights of the embryo independent from its social relations has been well documented in the ethnography of funerary rituals. These are reflected in many cultures in their association with different developmental stages of the embryo, for example, in traditional Hindu ceremonies for miscarriages during the fifth and the seventh month of pregnancy (Stevenson 1920: 113).[2] Legal history also shows us that the same is true for Western traditions, where causing the death of an animated embryo, for example, has also been categorised as murder (García Marín 1980). On the other hand, we also have to qualify the idea that new technologies and new scientific knowledge associated with reproduction place us in a post-relational world. It has been argued that precisely the opposite occurs in current processes of the geneticisation of the person and the increasing dissemination of genetic discourses. The medicalisation of family and kinship, as described by Kaja Finkler (2001), for example, is a good case in point. She shows how a person in certain clinical contexts is increasingly conceptualised through his or her relations with their ancestors. In the same line of thinking, much contemporary ethical discussion and legislation concerning the rights of the embryo present an image of the embryo that is different from the autonomous being depicted by some anthropologists. There is an ever-increasing emphasis placed on the highly valued cultural truth inscribed in the genetic combination that leads to a new human being. Thus, in the context of artificial insemination by donor (AID), as well as in the context of international adoption, the traditional view of giving involuntarily childless couples 'the right' to have a child is increasingly being displaced by 'the right' of every human being to have access to his or her genetic make-up. In order to be able to provide true genealogical stories for future sons and daughters, the expectation of anonymity of gamete donors is questioned, to the point that countries like Norway do not permit the donation of ova (see Melhuus and Howell, this volume). And the efforts deployed internationally by adopted individuals demanding access to their genetic origins translate a similar preoccupation in a different context (Legrand 2004).

We shall now attempt to make sense of the presence of the relational person in the present-day Western situation by returning to the topic of incest prohibition which has been central in the anthropological study of kinship. We adopt a historical and comparative perspective to reconsider the rupture that has been posited in Western kinship. Addressing the problem of how kinship is presently defined, we consider incest prohibitions in Western traditions, paying particular attention to the idioms in which these prohibitions are expressed. We also aim to analyse the relationship between kinship symbols, personal identity and kinship organisation.

Incest, Personhood and Relatedness

Sexual and matrimonial prohibitions are closely interrelated in the cultures with which we are concerned and they provide another perspective on kinship, making it possible to identify components that are found in each system. Key questions about the status of incest prohibitions in kinship require a cross-cultural perspective on sexual prohibitions. We argue that incest rules appear to be associated, at least partially, with native ideologies on personhood and relatedness.

Without doubt the work of Schneider constitutes a milestone in the history of the anthropology of kinship. His opposition between being and doing in the cultural definition of kinship, which is at the core of his later work on Yapese kinship, raises important questions about the overwhelming presence of the anthropologist's notions of kinship and the person when studying other cultures. Schneider proposes exercising epistemological vigilance, which echoes propositions already formulated by Arthur Hocart (1968) and Rodney Needham (1971), both of whom challenged the overemphasis placed on genealogy in the anthropological comprehension of non-Western categories of relatedness. While this is salutary, it seems to us that a radical position which denies any universality to the facts of what we call kinship constitutes a net loss to our understanding and indeed a very important one.

Schneider addressed sexual and matrimonial prohibitions among the Yapese in an early article (1957), but he developed his approach in a volume devoted to the subject of incest (1976). It was in the latter that he presented his culturalist views on the topic, making the important point that 'the most frequent confusion found in the literature in my experience is the confusion between the question of the origin of the prohibition on incest and the question of why it is maintained long after the conditions which may account for its origin have passed' (Schneider 1976: 156). He went on to argue that 'the incest prohibition is not universal', supporting this affirmation with the cases of brother–sister marriages of Pharaonic and Ptolemaic Egypt, the 'apparent lack' of an incest prohibition in ancient Iran, and the marriages between members of the royal family of Hawaii as analysed by Marshall Sahlins (Schneider 1976: 154). None of these relations would be considered as incestuous for the native people. He also insisted on the inclusion of kin other than nuclear kin in the different prohibitions that Europeans identify as incestuous, on the importance of elements such as food for determining who a person can and cannot have sexual relations with and on cases in which incest includes non-sexual behaviour. He then proposed equating incest with the idea of acting 'ungrammatically' in a given cultural code (Schneider 1976: 167). Thus, for Schneider, a priori definitions of incest based on a Western tendency to relate kinship to sexual intercourse and the birth of a child should be avoided. Rather, he argued, we should adopt a cultural and symbolic approach towards each case. But, in spite of these exhortations, he seems to have left the window open so that what he had previously excluded by closing the front door could re-enter. Reformulating ideas already put forward by Edmund Leach (1969) and Rodney Needham (1971), Schneider proposed a way forward for the anthropologist and argued for the possibility of comparison:

> The solution is really quite simple and is one used all the time: starting with the Western European cultural definition and then looking in each culture for something that is vaguely like it, then proceeding to identify the similarities and the differences, and by continuing to compare, expanding the horizon to the point where there are a series of different cultural definitions, a series of different cultural meanings and an array of various symbols for those meanings. (Schneider 1976: 160)

It is clear from this that not only can the Western reference not be eliminated from Schneider's analysis but also that it constitutes the bridge to other systems of thought. In fact, in the final part of his article, omitting even there to say that sexual prohibitions with genealogically related persons exist, Schneider returned to the cases that supposedly invalidate the universality of incest. By doing this, he curiously and implicitly accepted that 'blood is thicker than water', and not only in the West:

> For the royal Hawaiians, the Egyptians, for Samoa (as Shore describes the situation), for aristocratic twins in Bali (as Belo describes the situation), the problem is of maintaining the sacred qualities which are carried 'in the blood' so that they are not so dissipated as to lose their power, yet at the same time to maintain such ties with less sacred lines so that one line does not have a total monopoly of the royal, sacred quality. (Schneider 1976: 167)

But then, given the importance of this case for the critique of the notion of kinship, a legitimate question remains. What about the Yap?

In the same volume of the *Journal of Polynesian Society*, an analysis by David Labby on Yapese culture (Labby 1976) receives Schneider's approval.[3] The article reported that, among the Yap, biological sisters as well as a biological mother are strictly forbidden to any man as sexual partners. The biological daughter occupies a second level of prohibition. The Yap associate such sexual relations with endocannibalism and animality, which are expressed in idioms of embodiment. Images of 'blood' and land impregnated by the labour of ancestors are used to portray incest. These Yap idioms of incest, as well as the other examples presented by Schneider himself on the 'critical cases', in our opinion, show the universality of incest and oblige us to reconsider the radical critique of kinship that Schneider developed soon afterwards in *A Critique of the Study of Kinship*. Curiously enough, in this later work, he made the sociological argument that, among the Yap, genealogical positions are reliant on service and land relationships – a similar argument to that proposed earlier by Edmund Leach in Pul Eliya (Leach 1961). It could be argued that Schneider's culturalism and genealogical recall were selective.

From this point we confront the key question: on what are sexual prohibitions founded? Sexual and matrimonial rules normally appear to be associated with native ideologies about the person and relatedness (Héritier 1994). Consubstantiality, deriving from the transmission of body substance between generations or between the conjugal couple, or as a result of consuming the same foods (Jeudi-Ballini 1992; Carsten 1996), seems to occupy a central role here. This consubstantiality also occurs in inverse cases: for example, in the close marriages that are directed to preserve the qualities of the blood also cited by Schneider, and found among the Polynesian Tonga (Douaire-Marsaudon 2002). While still keeping in mind that kinship is not limited to this, it is worth retaining the idea that kinship is, at least, about consubstantiality.

From the problem of how kinship is defined anthropologically, we turn to incest prohibitions in Western traditions. It is through the prism of incest that we choose to approach Western kinship ideologies and in order to better understand a world in which 'blood is thicker than water'. Now we have established the fact that consubstantiality constitutes a bridge between European and other cultures, we may better focus on the possible discontinuities within European traditions. To be more precise, we shall explore the transition from blood to genes.[4]

Incest in Europe

In the history of Europe, the possibility of sex or marriage with kin has always been a source of anxiety. In the past, institutions regulating marriage persecuted those violating the more or less severe restrictions in the sexual and therefore the matrimonial arena. The same anxieties were expressed by individuals, as can be seen in the case of a woman well known through the historical work of Le Roy Ladurie. This woman declared in front of the Inquisition that she refused a man as a lover because she had previously had sex with his cousin (Le Roy Ladurie 1980: 150). Her fear goes beyond the strict framework of marriage prohibitions.

Before the Reformation, prohibitions in Christian Europe reached limits that are now difficult to imagine – up to the eighth canonical degree (the equivalent to the genealogical position of FFFFFFFBSSSSSSch) – particularly if we consider that the prohibitions concerned small and endogamous local peasant communities. What is perhaps even more difficult for us to grasp is that prohibitions normally went up to the same limit for the consanguines of ego's deceased partner (the affines). This was justified by the canonical idea that, through sexual intercourse, husband and wife became 'one flesh' (Porqueres i Gené 2000). Other prohibitions were also in place, for example, deriving from a promise of marriage and related to the consanguineous kin of the *sponsa* or *sponsus* (the engaged couple), as well as those deriving from godparenthood.

Most of these prohibitions have now disappeared. Such a reduction is part of a general trend across Europe that has continued since the beginning of the twentieth century. In England, for example, marriage with the sister of a deceased wife was allowed in 1907, and marriage with the brother of a deceased husband in 1921. Nowadays, the Catholic Church Canon Law (code of 1983) only maintains restrictions up to consanguineous cousins (Canon 1091) and uniquely for in-laws' lineal kin (Canon 1092) and also with lineal kin and up to brother and sister in adoption (Canon 1094). Canon 1093 upholds the impediment of public propriety that 'arises when a couple lives together after an invalid marriage, or from a notorious or public concubinage'. It invalidates marriage between a man or a woman and his/her spouse's lineal kin (in the first degree and vice versa). The point to underline here is that prohibitions deriving from repeated sexual relations, via concubinage, are more extensive in the code of 1917 than in the code of 1983. In 1917, the notion of public propriety 'invalidates a living marriage in the first and second degree of the direct line between the man and the blood relatives of the woman, and vice versa'. All this seems to confirm that sexual and matrimonial prohibitions are concentrated in consanguinity, if we leave aside the prohibitions derived from the commingling of husband and wife through sexual intercourse – an idea strong in England, for instance, up to the beginning of the twentieth century, as Adam Kuper (2002) has recently reminded us. The physical bond in kinship becomes exclusively and more and more transparently (but without suppressing the 'one flesh' bond) as 'being of the same blood' (see Wolfram 1987).

It is worth considering the reasons for these prohibitions in their historical sequence. First, why should one not have sexual relations with or marry a consanguine? Before the nineteenth century, incest prohibitions were explained by the respect due to relatives, by the need to create ties between families through marriage, by the necessity of avoiding the concurrence in the same person of more than one genealogical position, by the sexual indifference created by a common residence and, more or less explicitly, by the link of physical sameness or shared physical substance – which explains not only the prohibitions between blood relatives but also between those linked by marriage or sexual intercourse. During the nineteenth century, with the advances in scientific research on human evolution and heredity, the prohibition of incest increasingly acquired a biomedical justification: children born from a marriage between close kin, it was said, frequently suffer from some kind of malformation. The emergence of genetics as a science provided a scientific base for these considerations and, today, incest prohibitions are spontaneously justified by genetics: marriages among close relatives, where there is a high genetic correlation, would aggravate, it is said, the risk of genetic disease or disorder.

The risk of marrying a first cousin was greatly debated in England at the end of nineteenth century and the debate had parliamentary implications. Important scholars, such as Maine, Westermark, Lubbock and even Darwin, who, like Maine, married his first cousin, participated in the elaboration of arguments and statistics that were eventually used to conclude that there was no danger in first-cousin marriage. In the United States, the outcome of the discussion was different and led to the institutionalisation of the prohibition of marriage between cousins in a number of states and, as Kuper suggests, to the institutionalisation and justification of eugenics. In the Catholic world, the question of nature became central in nineteenth century Catholic theology. This was marked by so-called Neothomism, which tended to naturalise social hierarchies. Thus, following the publication of the Code of 1917, the important *Dictionnaire de Théologie Catholique* was to add, in the 1920s, for the first time, a purely genetic argument for justifying matrimonial prohibitions between consanguineous kin. First, unions with ascendants and descendants were forbidden because of natural law. Then, the prohibition concerning collaterals was justified: 'because of the classic respect due to consanguines and because of the nature of the affection that has to unite them; because of the need of not tapering charity inside too narrow limits; because of the danger of physical malformations resulting for the children of those unions' (Cimelier 1932: 1997).

The legal reasoning that supports the prohibitions of the Hungarian civil code is not, in fact, very far removed from these Catholic arguments. To start with, the Hungarian code also makes a distinction between lineal and collateral kin. Whilst intercourse between siblings, considered a misdemeanour, is punishable with up to two years imprisonment, the code sanctions as a felony both sexual intercourse (*közösülés*) and other sexual relations (*fajtalanság*) between lineal descendants (for example, grandfather, father, child, etc.), with up to five years of imprisonment unless the descendant engaged in such a felony is a minor, which would add the crime of sexual abuse. The official legal policy behind the definition of these crimes is the protection of a 'healthy lineage' and the 'security' of blood ties, both subsumed under the common label of endangering society. (According to the Hungarian criminal law, in order to qualify an act as a misdemeanour or felony, the act, *inter alia*, would endanger society.)

The preoccupation with consanguinity in sexual intercourse continues up to the present, and frequently goes far beyond what is considered scientifically rational. Such is the case in Austria, where several women requested to be fertilised by the frozen semen found inside Ötzi, a hunter who had lived during the fourth millennium BC and was preserved in a glacier in the Alps. The argument to legitimise the refusal recalls the special place of lineal kin in the economy of incest: 'The authorities are embarrassed and finally refuse the request: Ötzi could be the ancestor of the volunteer, and in this case there would be union in the direct line, incest in spite of the millenaries' (Poly 2003: 9). The same fear surfaces in the regulations concerning artificial insemination by donor (AID). Already the English Warnock Report, opening the door to the possibility of 'incest' in affinity (a brother of the husband may give his sperm to his sister-in-law in a private arrangement), had recommended reducing the number of children fathered by a single donor. This was in order to minimise 'the risk of passing on a recessive condition' and, in addition, even if 'the true medical and genetic consequences of inadvertent incest or marriage within the prohibited degrees are often over-stated', such a recommendation was needed in order to face the 'fear consistently expressed ... that AID children may unwittingly enter into an incestuous relationship or contract a marriage within the prohibited degrees' (Warnock 1985: 22, 25–26). Thus, it recommended that any single donor should father a maximum of ten children, and by analogy the same should apply to egg donors. Rabbinic authorities in Israel go even further: here the fear of incest justifies the prohibition of any insemination using sperm from an anonymous Jewish donor (Kahn 2000: 97).

In 1985, a special commission of the Spanish Parliament debated AID and *in vitro* fertilisation. The same need to regulate the number of times any one sperm donor can become a 'father' was extensively discussed. The argument about the danger to the offspring coming from eventual incestuous relationships kept resurfacing. For Spanish biologists and geneticists, it appeared to be necessary to limit the number of pregnancies that derive from the same donor in a given territory. The argument revolved on the risk of consanguineous incest, which increases the possibility of recessive gene disorders. Taking an extreme position, Professor Lacadena Calero concluded strikingly: 'The consequence is that incest is genetically bad.' Expounding on his statement, and after recognising the low chances of 'genetic incest' resulting from AID, he expressed his fears on the matter in this way: 'It is said that these things are charged by the devil; even if one would wish things to be otherwise, it doesn't stop a person marrying a sister or a half-brother, taking things to this extreme.' Later he proposed that as a solution donors should only be allowed to donate once and further that only one embryo resulting from a sperm donation should be allowed. During the same parliamentary debate, Canon Law Professor M. Souto, after recalling the traditional explanations for prohibiting incest, adopted a similar argument and used the authority of science to support his case. He argued that, given the 'natural' risk that effectively exists, any kind of donation should be banned – because there is always the possibility of a donor having sexual relations with his own daughter.

Certainly, the phantasms of consanguineous incest are present in the field of genetics and particularly in AID. This also appears among potential users of the technologies, as Edwards has shown in a recent article that focuses on such issues in England (Edwards 2004). In the same vein, French couples seeking to have a baby through AID or embryo transfer are travelling to Spain, where they can obtain embryos or gametes that are obviously not related to them. There is evidence that some are refusing frozen embryos offered to them in France because of the fear that their future child might have a sexual relationship with his or her genetic sibling in the future.[5] But we should return to more formal examples. In Australia, legal measures have existed since 1983 that reflect a preoccupation with consanguinity and incest. In that year, the South Australian Code of Practice prevented the use of reproductive material when: (1) a woman's ovum was used with the sperm of her father, son, brother or half-brother; and (2) a man's sperm was used with the ovum of mother, daughter, sister or half-sister.

In February 2003, the Australian Health Ethics Committee produced a draft report for public consultation called Guidelines on the Use of Reproductive Technology in Clinical Practice and Research. This report raised another kind of preoccupation concerning AID with closely related donors. The document points first to the fact that 'use of relatives of the recipients as gamete donors raises a number of serious issues, including the complexity of long-term family arrangements, the potential for coercion of the gamete donors, and possible psychosexual consequences for all participants and their spouses and partners'. Secondly, it claims 'that oocytes should not be fertilised (whether *in vivo* or *in vitro*) with sperm from a close genetic relative of the female gamete provider, that is, from a person for whom a sexual relationship to the oocyte provider would legally be considered to be incest'.

We see here a two-pronged statement about the inconvenience of closely related donors in AID. Apart from a preoccupation with avoiding close genetic relatives (the Australian laws include in the category of incest all lineal kin as well as siblings), expressed without any kind of explanation, there is also reference to a set of problems that, in accordance with the economy of the text, seems to concern more distant kin, including affines. When more distant kin appear as potential gamete donors, three different non-exhaustive arguments are provided, each of them having to do with the internal relations of the family and, mainly, with order within the family. Actually, 'the complexity of long-term family arrangements and the psychosexual consequences for all participants and their spouses and partners' seems to acquire its full meaning if we consider these problems in the light of phrases such as 'a healthy lineage' and 'the security of the blood tie', which were at the centre of the Hungarian legislation concerning the prohibition of incest. In fact, with this argument we find ourselves in a familiar landscape, namely the crucial importance of avoiding the conflation of genealogical kin positions through the sexual union of close kin. It would seem that arguments about the necessity of maintaining the discreteness of kinship terms, which goes back to ancient Greece and proceeds through the Canon Laws on marriage, still have currency today. These findings show that in a hyper-scientific context, the issue of incest, directly linked to the definition of the family and the person, is still informed by metaphysical considerations.

Clearly, more than a physical dimension is present in the domain of kinship. The irreducibility of the individual, which certain scholars nowadays relate to the chance combination of genetic material coming from 'both sides', echoes traditional histories of individualisation through the acquisition of a unique soul for the embryo at a particular moment during its development. Nevertheless, in spite of strong continuities, which we believe are underestimated by some anthropologists, it is clear that during the last century the increasing prominence of a genetic paradigm has meant that genes have become an essential symbol of kinship and identity.[6] New definitions are thus surfacing. The father, for example, is no longer *'quem nuptiae demonstrant'*, but *'quem sanguis demonstrat'*. We are also witnessing another major tendency, in that recognition of the lineal transmission of biogenetic substance is becoming increasingly dominant to the exclusion of the recognition of affinal transmission. The physical bond in kinship is increasingly becoming about 'having the same genes' in a way that is exclusive. For a biologist, for example, kinsmen may be relatives through filiation but not through marriage. But, here again, some nuance is required.

Incest, Telegony and *Una Caro*

As already noted, the recent concentration of sexual and matrimonial prohibitions in consanguinity is displacing prohibitions traditionally derived from the idea of the commingling of husband and wife through sexual intercourse – an idea that was at the centre of the cognatic kinship system created by the Christian Church and exported to family law adopted in different countries. This representation, dating from antiquity, is a throw back to the injunction in Genesis that impelled men to abandon their father and mother in order to become one flesh (*una caro*) with their wife: 'For this cause shall a man leave his father and mother, and shall cleave to his wife, and they shall be two in one flesh.' Christians, through the Epistles of Saint Paul, but also the Talmud of the same period, take seriously the idea that through sex husband and wife become 'one flesh'.

Such developments induce an increasing symmetry in the prohibitions, concluding not only in complete bilateralism but in the complete parallelism between consanguineal and affinal positions. Just as the Church and Christ became one body through their mystical union, so also marriage, in its secular image, makes two bodies one through sexual intercourse. If ego becomes one flesh with his or her partner, then logically the blood relatives of the partner become blood relatives of ego and vice versa. This is the explicit logic of the affinal prohibition put forward progressively by Christianity in the first centuries AD. Later, the focus of legislation would directly mention sex relations explicitly considered to be the vector of the transformations that the husband and wife have undergone. The result was to be the prohibitions called *ex affinitas superveniens* and *ex copula illicita*, which forbade any sexual or marital link with the consanguineous kin of a lover and with the lover of a consanguine. These persisted up to the twentieth century when they were partially reformulated in the prohibitions of 'public property', already mentioned. Thus, in earlier periods of European history, natural identity as the sharing of substances is not simply defined among ascendants and descendants but also among spouses and among relations by sex.[7] This idea is by no means specific to Christian and Jewish traditions, as Héritier shows in her work on 'incest of the second type' (Héritier 1994).

It is important to underline that there is a particularly persistent belief associated with the configuration we have presented. Telegony, or the theory of impregnation, rests on the idea that a woman can give birth to children resembling not only her current partner, but also to one or more preceding sexual partners; the hereditary characteristics of a man are thus believed to 'impregnate' the matrix of his partner and are later passed on to her children, whoever their genetic father may be. For the majority of the authors writing on this topic, the woman would first have to become pregnant, but some consider that sexual intercourse itself is sufficient. In this context, nineteenth-century biologists passionately discussed the case of a mare that had been 'impregnated' by a zebra and had given birth to a foal with streaked paws, while its mate was a magnificent Arab stallion (de Varigny 1897; Cousin 1904). In 1931, a French doctor, Selbonne, wrote a medical thesis that was favourable to this theory and mentioned that, during the First World War, women raped by Germans refused to have children for fear of this impregnation.

Edouard Conte and Cornelia Essner (1995) undertook a detailed study of the consequences of this belief for the racial theories shared by German nationalists from the end of the nineteenth century until the Second World War. For the influential anti-Semitic ideologist J. Streicher, for example, sexual intercourse with a Jewish man resulted in the woman being unable to give birth to Aryan offspring. The argument was that 'male sperm, during the sexual act, is absorbed completely or partly by the maternal matter and so passes into the blood. A single sexual intercourse of a Jew with an Aryan woman is enough for poisoning the blood of the latter for ever' (Conte and Essner 1995: 131).

Telegony is no longer taken seriously, and recurrent considerations of the possibility of recourse to in-laws in the domain of new techniques of medically assisted reproduction indicate a change in the status of the 'one flesh' theory.[8] In any case, it is important to stress here that the relational character of alliance remains on the agenda in defining the genetic tie, as well as in the implementation of the new techniques of reproduction. In both scientific and lay representations, in spite of the lack of necessity of either sexual relations or marriage in new reproductive technologies, the union of a male and a female gamete constitutes the necessary basis for any genetic link to be formed. This occurs in an ordinary genealogical way or by jumping two generations as in the case of cloning where the nucleus of the cell of the cloned person reverts back to his or her father and mother as the providers of genetic information. In addition, the perturbations evoked by certain normative texts that discuss 'the complexity of long-term family arrangements' as potentially dangerous to stability within the family are worth examining. Both the 'security of the blood tie' and disputes over authority and privileged links to the baby are present in the ethnography. Kin who have more than one genealogical position and couples having to rely on kin in order to conceive a child, as well as the new relations facing gamete donors with new relatives, are all strong reminders that the child is not completely the child of the social father or mother. Commenting on discussions between English women on this topic, Edwards remarks: 'A person is a mother if she provides an ovum, and an aunt if she is the mother's sister: what happens if she is both? If you were to donate an egg to your sister, these women point out, you might have a stake in the ensuing child that would compel you to interfere in its upbringing' (Edwards 2004: 762–63). In the same vein, obtaining semen from the husband's father also bothers, Edwards continues: 'Lyndsay asks all of us present to imagine using your "boyfriend's dad's sperm … It would feel like you had sex with your boyfriend's father … The baby would be like your boyfriend's brother"' (Edwards 2004: 763). Certainly, here affinity appears to matter.

Undoubtedly, this kind of representation lacks the social impact of those stressing the genetic link between the gamete donor and the receiver. These conceptions do not seem to have the same influence everywhere. For the most part, formal incest prohibitions focus explicitly on genetic parenthood, leaving aside affinal or even strictly biological parenthood. Even if relativisation of the genetic and the biological maternal link is possible and indeed current in the context of NRT (Bestard 2004b), an interesting asymmetry emerges when considering incest. What is possible in one case appears impossible in another. In this context, Charis Thompson's (2001) examination of Californian infertility clinics is particularly instructive. In her examples, a surrogate mother can be the sister of the man whose sperm conceives the baby she carries. Still more interestingly, one such surrogate mother said she was happy to have had her Fallopian tubes 'tied' impeding any possibility of becoming the genetic mother of the baby and she saw her role as just an ancillary one, since everyone accepts that in no way is she contributing to the 'baby's nature'.

In any case, discontinuities between the pre-genetic and the genetic paradigms are not always self-evident. In some cases, a focus on genetic material provokes statements to the effect that the arrival of the gene on the scene eliminates biological arguments. Scientific conceptions of incest have little to do with the sharing of biological substance. But blood seems to still have its place. In the context of surrogate motherhood, however, scientific considerations of the transmission of biogenetic characteristics from a surrogate mother to the child they agree to carry are echoed in lay discourse. The link generated between a surrogate mother and fetus through the blood they share also feeds the fear of the possibility that two persons, without genetic ties, but born from the same surrogate mother, might later commit incest (Edwards 2004).

Nowadays, the meanings of 'blood' and 'genes' tend to be separated but there are ways in which both terms are used that make their meanings similar or even equivalent. Does this justify our own starting point of affirming the validity of a 'substantive paradigm' for kinship in order to explore the contemporary context? Up to what point can we treat genetic transmission, conceptualised purely as a combination of information, as being a transmission of a substance? In fact, from the historical materials we have been working with, the opposite question arises – up to what point is the transmission of blood and substance strictly understandable from a substantive approach? Blood, mainly that of the father, also seems to operate as a programmer, as is clearly evident in the influential vision of Aristotle, and we should not forget that the opposition between form and matter is central in European representations of reproduction. For Aristotle, gestation is above all a *trophè* (the mother feeds the embryo) and thus reproduction is conceived as the result of the male active role (the fertilising principle) and the female passive role (the feeder principle). Aristotle uses the analogy of the potter with the clay or the carpenter with the wood to demonstrate such social constructions of reproduction.[9] The man gives shape while woman gives matter. In spite of that, as in the classical Canon Law model of the transmission of the blood of the father and the mother to the child, the father's blood is depicted in substantive terms, although there is no accepted notion of the substantive contribution of semen to the formation and nourishment of the fetus during intrauterine life through repeated sexual relations.[10] The idea of semen as a source of energy and a purely informational germ line seems to have existed in the past, thus making traditional references to blood closer to current references to genes than is sometimes recognised (Sissa 1989). In any case, in both pre-genetic and genetic contexts substances physically support the agent that makes the encounter with the partner and thus the procreative process possible.

As well as the opposition between form and matter – certainly of lesser importance in the predominant Hippocratic and Galenic bilateral embryogenetic systems – the active/passive opposition has also played a significant part in representations of reproduction. We can still see this today, not only in the popular imagination, but also in scientific discourse (Martin 1991; Héritier 1996; Konrad 1998). Could this opposition explain some of the asymmetries observed in the meanings assigned to sperm and ova within the process of reproduction? Or in their respective moral value? Even if this opposition is not always explicit, this issue merits further exploration.

Conclusion

There is no doubt that relationality, albeit associated with an overemphasis on the individual, is central to the contemporary situation. If some anthropologists have decided to treat the current epoch as exceptional and have pointed to a strictly new individualistic orientation, re-examining the classic anthropological issue of incest leads us to conclude that there is an important degree of continuity between the past and the present and between Western and non-Western kinship systems. We hope through our chapter to contribute to building a bridge between the analysis of our own occidental kinship reality and other realities in the world without diminishing what, in our view, is the priority of the body. We argue that the body is the lowest common denominator of every kinship system. Keeping in mind that kinship is not only this, it is worth recalling that recent studies show that all cultures (even the ones supposedly giving greater place to practice) express connections between relatives through some kind of 'consubstantiality'. This consubstantiality is created by the transmission of bodily characteristics between generations or between the conjugal couple, or is created through food.[11] Since genes can be said not to be 'substances', this has opened up the possibility of a radical rupture between the contemporary Western situation and the past and between Western and non-Western. We have argued that, while there are important ruptures, there are also equally strong continuities. Thus, in the domains of genes and blood, we have identified equivalences between the treatment of blood and genes in discourses surrounding incest prohibition. We have argued that traditional conceptualisations of blood – as well as known metaphors connected to 'seeds', which act as information devices in the field of procreation (Delaney 1991) – are not fundamentally different from the communicational character of genetic transmission. Blood was a programmer in Aristotelian and Galenic models of conception prior to the emergence of genetics. From there, instead of radically questioning the consubstantialist approach to kinship, we think it worth enlarging by subsuming it into a more general embodiment paradigm. In our opinion, the evidence that a crucial part of the relations described in universal incest prohibitions is inscribed in the body of related persons opens the possibility of a better understanding of kinship, wherever it is.

Notes

1. In a subsequent paper, the author is particularly clear when dealing with the non-necessity of the social relations arising from mere procreation: 'the facts of procreation that establish kinship refer to a physical process that, beyond telling us that the act also creates a relationship between creator and created, is neutral as to the nature of that relationship' (Strathern 1995: 354).
2. Thus, leaving aside the current burial ceremonies for fetuses in Parisian hospitals (information kindly given by Marika Moisseeff), the Tamils studied by Reynolds consider that the embryo is only alive from the second trimester inside the womb, but with a kind of non-autonomous life. If there is miscarriage about the fourth or the fifth month of pregnancy, the rituals for delivery and birth pollution are observed but not those of death (Reynolds 1978: 128).
3. See also Schneider (1957: 791): 'The incest taboo on Yap applies to members of the nuclear family, the patrilineal lineage and the matrilineal clan. The prohibition on sexual relations among members of these groups applies to all and any, regardless of genealogical distance.'
4. We thank Julia Ribot, Judit Sándor and Ildikó Takács for the information they kindly gave us on the Spanish and the Hungarian contexts.
5. Personal communication from Geneviève Delaisi de Parseval, clinician.
6. The emphasis on the increasing trend towards individualism is ceding to a growing interest in the relational nature of genes, and their social impact. Thus, Siebert (1995), in an article quoted by Finkler (2001), wrote: 'Genes are suddenly thought to be responsible for everything from poverty to privilege, from misdemeanors to murder. I seem to recall watching television one night and seeing a man up on homicide charges offer as defense the presence of a "criminal gene", which he claimed ran in his family.' This certainly constitutes a good example of the contemporary over-geneticisation of behaviours. Nevertheless, here again, it is useful to recall that we can retrace such anecdotes back to Aristotle, who described how a court acquitted a man who had struck his father, because he was able to prove that his father had behaved in the same way; the fault, Aristotle tells us, was thus seen as natural and nobody could consequently reproach him; see *Magna Moralia*, II, 6, 20, 1202.
7. People have used this legal definition. Besides the example of Le Roy Ladurie already cited, it is interesting to note that in France in the fourteenth century, families trying to impede a non-desired marriage of a child claimed previous sexual relations between the undesired partner and a close relative of the child (Flandrin 1981: 77).
8. Except apparently for some animal breeders, who continue to defend such ideas.
9. See Aristotle (1979) *Generation of Animals* 1.22, 730b5–6ff. See the recent work of Bonnard (2004).
10. A common idea in many other contexts, in Africa and also in Oceania (Godelier 2004).
11. See, for example, the works of Janet Carsten, Monique Jeudi-Ballini, Andrew Strathern.

CHAPTER 8

'LOVING MOTHERS' AT WORK: RAISING OTHERS' CHILDREN AND BUILDING FAMILIES WITH THE INTENTION TO LOVE AND TAKE CARE

Enikő Demény

Introduction

There is a well-known saying in Hungary, *'anya csak egy van'* ('there is only one mother'), which is meant to express the exceptional value given to mothers. However, there are life situations when this saying is not true. For example, for the four-year-old boy who lives in the SOS Children's Village in Kecskemét, Hungary, it is the most 'natural' thing in the world that he has two mothers. As the little boy himself expressed it, he has one 'birth mother' ('szülő anya') and one 'loving mother' ('szerető anya'). The 'loving mother' is an innovative term used to name his foster-mother and has been 'created' by this little boy to make sense of the realities of his life. His birth mother gave birth to nine children and all of them were left by her immediately after birth at the hospital, in the same way as the birth mother was herself left in the hospital by her own mother years before. The boy was placed in an orphanage and later on he was taken to the SOS Children's Village. In the imagination of this small boy it is normal that one mother gives birth to children, and another mother finds these children and will love and raise them. However, not all children who are not raised by their biological mothers can say that they have a 'loving mother'. In Hungary there are many children who grow up in orphanages or in other types of institutional childcare settings where they do not have a 'mother'. Children who are raised in SOS Children's Villages are given a 'mother' who is responsible for their care and whom they can relate to. These mothers are women who work as full-time professional foster-mothers and are employed by the SOS Children's Village organisation.

The first SOS Children's Village was set up in 1949 in the Austrian Tyrol. The founder of the organisation, Hermann Gmeiner, realised that the Second World War had left behind, on the one hand, many orphans and, on the other, many widows and single women without children. His main idea was to bring them together and in this way to offer orphan children a mother and a family. Taking into account that all over the world there are many orphans or abandoned children and a number of women who would like to raise children, it is not surprising that the SOS Children's Village initiative became an international organisation. Currently there are more than one thousand SOS villages in more than a hundred countries on five continents.

The SOS Children's Village's family model is based on the figure of the foster-mother. Beside the figure of the mother, three other principles shape the ideology of the village: the brotherhood between brothers and sisters, the family house and the village. One of the often mentioned strengths of the SOS Village model is the possibility for siblings to grow up together, in contrast with some other types of childcare institutions, where they are often separated based on their age or gender.

The SOS mothers raise five to eight children in the family houses provided by the organisation. There are certain minimum standards for the professional profile of these mothers. According to these standards, a future SOS mother has to be aged between twenty-five and forty, she has to be single, widowed, divorced or separated and has to be in good physical and mental health. The SOS mothers are not prohibited from having a male partner, but they are required to live alone in the village (Gmeiner 1993: 27–47). It is up to them, however, how they spend their spare time outside the village. The SOS mothers may have their own older or adult children and in some cases SOS mothers are allowed to take their younger children with them to the SOS Children's Village, but this is not common practice.

In addition to the already mentioned criteria, there are numerous others that should also be met by an SOS mother. According to the job advertisements, the SOS mother should be resilient, patient, capable of building relationships, willing to learn, practical minded, independent, self-confident and good-natured. Furthermore she has to be prepared to get involved with children who in some cases face severe mental and emotional problems, and to deal with them in a loving and supporting way. To find out whether a candidate meets not only the formal, but also the additional desired criteria, she has to spend a period of practical training in the SOS Children's Village, working as a helping mother. The aim of this period is to enable both parties, the SOS Children's Village organisation as well as the SOS mother candidate, to come to a suitable decision. Following the selection procedure, the SOS mother candidates receive theoretical and practical training in preparation for their future tasks.

The SOS mothers receive a salary for their work. Beside this, they get an allowance for the housekeeping expenses as well as for those connected with the children's needs. The mothers' duty is to take care of children, to keep the house and to keep account of the money they use. The head of the village and the educationalist (both of them are usually men) have to live in the village together with their own families. They are not only indirectly the employers of the mothers but also in accordance with the ideology of the SOS Children's Village organisation, they provide the 'paternal element' for the children. The other male employees of the village, the gardener, the village master and the driver, have the same 'duty'. Therefore beside their daily job, they are supposed to act as male role models for the children (Gmeiner 1993: 48–54).[1]

Identity and Relatedness, Discourse and Practice

This chapter is based on anthropological fieldwork carried out in the SOS Children's Village in Kecskemét, Hungary, where I conducted in-depth interviews with women who are working there as full-time, professional foster-mothers.[2] The purpose of my research was to get an insight into how professional foster-mothers in this SOS Children's Village construct, define and represent their identity as social foster mothers in relation to the dominant social, legal, and institutional 'discourses' connected with family, motherhood, relatedness and women's roles in society.[3] Through the analysis of the SOS mothers' narratives, my intention was to make visible how the naturalised and taken for granted realities about family and motherhood affect the lives of those particular subjects who occupy a marginal position in connection with the dominant discourses of family and relatedness. Although I was focusing on identity politics of professional foster-mothers, during fieldwork it became more and more clear that family and kinship thinking also has relevance in such institutionalised contexts. Taking into account that anthropological studies of kinship and family were not traditionally carried out in such kinds of institutional settings, my analysis can offer a view on how ideas about relatedness and family are employed in these contexts.

In the course of her/his life, each person develops a personal image of the family. This image (called social representation in social psychology) on the one hand, incorporates the individual's personal experiences and, on the other, is derived from information and thought patterns received and passed on as traditions in the course of education and social communication and interaction. It is an image that helps us to classify conditions, circumstances, phenomena and persons we come across, and the 'theories' that we can rely on (Moscovici 1995: 75–83). According to Foucault, the most authoritative systems of classification are those that are taken as natural rather than constructed, the 'Other' being incorporated into 'a natural order of disorder' (Foucault 1981: 44). Analysing the social representations of foster-motherhood and of the family of foster-mothers is useful in understanding how the traditional family concept developed in the course of socialisation is extended and transmitted by different institutional forms and by the subjects' own life experience. It can also give us an insight into how dominant ideologies about motherhood, family and women's role in society shape the meanings that are attributed by these professional foster-mothers to different types of relatedness (genetic, biological and social).

According to Henrietta Moore, self-identity is established socially through a set of discourses that is both discursive and practical and which establishes the grounds for identity and the framework(s) within which identity becomes intelligible. There is a potential discrepancy between a set of discourses that is culturally available and the individual experience, interpretation and understanding of those discourses (Moore 1994: 53–58). Women come to have different understandings of themselves as mothers because they are differently positioned with regard to dominant narratives concerning motherhood, and take up different positions in those narratives. An interesting question is what accounts for the differences between women with regard to their self-representations as engendered individuals and as mothers.

Naming is also central to questions of identity. To name something means also to define an identity, while to ascribe characteristics to that identity is an aspect of political power (Foucault 1981; Ricoeur 1992:149). It is political because it will always have material consequences. I draw on Foucault's ideas on the power to name in analysing the consequences of the fact that the women working in the SOS Village are called 'mothers'. The differentiation of social identities is also connected with the exercise of power. It is on the basis of the naturalised differences between these identities that the rights and needs of particular individuals are established. Rights and needs are differentially distributed between different sorts of persons and the ability to define a social identity is the ability to ascribe appropriate rights and needs (Moore 1994: 57). I shall argue in this chapter that both naming and ascription of rights and needs have particular relevance in understanding discourses related to professional foster-motherhood in Kecskemét.

There has been a tendency in anthropology to see mothers and the mother-child unit as having a universal function. This approach encourages the view that domestic units everywhere have the same form and function, which are dictated by the biological facts of reproduction and the necessity of child maintenance. Feminist critiques directly addressed this self-evident quality and the naturalness of motherhood and stressed that the concept of mother is not merely given in natural processes of pregnancy, birth or lactation, but is a cultural construction that different societies build up and elaborate in different ways (Thorne and Yalom 1992: 3–23). Therefore it is important not only to pay attention to the culturally diverse ways in which women perform their roles as mothers, but also to see how the category of women and the attitudes towards them are linked to ideas about marriage, family, home, children and work. Schweitzer notes that one of the problems with classic kinship studies is that by privileging the domain of kinship they separate it from the totality of social relations. He also points out that feminist interventions played an important role in highlighting the inseparable links among the social fields of gender, kinship, religion and economy (Schweitzer 2000: 214). In my analysis of foster-motherhood, I also emphasise that people act not as detached from social discourse but as part of it. My aim is to understand and represent socially constructed knowledge about what it means to be a foster-mother in a specific social environment and for specific subjects and to interpret these representations.

The production of knowledge by discursive practices is a process through which power hierarchies are constructed, maintained and challenged in the social sphere of subjects living under particular historical circumstances. By disclosing the experiences of mothers who occupy marginal positions in connection with the dominant narratives about family and relatedness, we can point out how the discursive and practical attempt to maintain the status quo regarding the 'normal' structure of the family affects the lives of those people who at a certain point in their life history end up living in a different, alternative setting. In addition, we can observe how boundaries between people are not only constructed alongside categories like class, ethnicity or gender but also created through following different life strategies. I shall argue, in line with Foucault (1998: 51), that discourses not only are cognitive constructs 'out there', but have powerful effects on people's lives.

The Social, Legal and Institutional Context of Foster-parenthood in Hungary

The dominant representations of motherhood in Hungary are linked to notions of the family, which represents a very important value for Hungarians. Surveys and opinion polls carried out during the last two decades show that for the majority of Hungarians the family is still the most important value in their lives; it is more important than any other area, such as work, friends or leisure.[4] According to various studies, the modern nuclear family, with a husband, a wife and their children still represents the 'ideal' family for the majority of Hungarians (Neményi 1995: 250–52, 2000; Lévai 2000: 185). Single parenthood is not considered an 'ideal' solution. (Kapitány 2003: 257–58). Ideas of women and motherhood are strongly correlated. Almost 95 per cent of the Hungarian respondents (both male and female) of the World Value Survey carried out in 1999 agreed with the statement 'women need children', while only 33 per cent of them agreed that 'men need children'.[5] In Hungary people do not think positively about remaining childless. Seventy per cent of the population reported that it is bad or very bad if there are no children in the family (Pongrácz and Molnár 1997: 97).

The current realities of the Hungarian family, however, differ from the ideal image of it. During the last quarter of the last century the Hungarian family underwent rapid change. The number of cohabiting couples with children and the number of single-headed households are increasing. The positive attitude towards children is less and less reflected in the actual practice of having children.[6]

The number of children raised in institutions in Hungary is high and many of them cannot be adopted.[7] The main aim of the child protection system is to integrate or reintegrate these children into their biological family. For those children for whom this integration or reintegration is not possible, the law intends to assure a 'family-like environment'. In order to achieve this aim it prescribes the deinstitutionalisation of the child care system for abandoned or orphan children and offers two possibilities for doing this. A first possibility is to fragment the already existing, huge and depersonalised childcare institutions and to transform them into so-called 'child homes' where no more then forty children are raised together. The second possibility is foster-care. The Child Protection Act of 1997 establishes the legal framework for a professional foster-parent network. While according to previous regulations only married couples were allowed to be foster-parents, the Act on Child Protection no longer connects this activity with the marital status or the gender of the candidate.[8] The condition to become a foster-parent is to attend and successfully pass the professional training required by law. By this means foster parenting has become a legally recognised profession in Hungary.

However, there are not many couples or persons in Hungary who would like to become foster-parents and raise the children of 'others', and the number of those who will assume the responsibility of raising children with disabilities is even smaller. In these conditions, many orphan or abandoned children are growing up in institutions. One would think that in these circumstances Hungarian society would realise the importance and value of the SOS foster-mothers' work, as the majority of the children raised by these mother do. The spontaneous remark of a five-year-old boy to his SOS foster-mother, 'Mom, it is so good that you were born for me', expresses how important the existence of the foster-mother and the care they bestow is to the children they raise. However, though it may seem surprising, instead of being appreciated for their work, the SOS foster-mothers are often labelled as deviant, and the SOS Children's Village organisation has been blamed in public discourses for creating incomplete families. While being a mother is highly valued in Hungary, being an SOS foster-mother is often looked upon with suspicion, or at least this is the feeling and the experience of those SOS mothers I came to know at the SOS Village in Kecskemét.

Living in an 'Incomplete Family'

Due to their particular social position, the women working as foster-mothers in the SOS Children's Village have to interpret and reinterpret the cultural meanings that are linked to motherhood in order to define their identity. This reinterpretation takes place along two main axes. First, these women have to construct, define and legitimise their identity as single women and single mothers in the framework of an institution – the SOS Children's Village – that is different from marriage. Secondly, they have to position themselves in the discourse about the biological and social aspects of motherhood and to interpret their mothering not (just) as an innate duty (or maternal instinct) but also as an acquired skill and a profession.

The SOS Children's Village organisation is often blamed in different public forums for creating 'incomplete' families. It is not difficult to guess that it is the 'ideal' image of the nuclear family that the SOS families are compared with, and that it is exactly this comparison that leads to the verdict 'incomplete'. Two main problems are identified in connection with these families. The first is the women's 'lack of a male partner' and the second is the children's 'lack of a father'. Due to these 'deviations' from the norm of the nuclear family, the activity of the SOS organisation and the work of the SOS mothers are very often looked upon with doubt and disapproval. Even their mothering abilities are questioned and they quite often have to face questions such as how they can be good mothers if they are not living with a male partner, in which case their sexual life is not 'balanced'.

The women's struggles with what it means to be a single 'mother' to the children they raise are shaped by the exclusions and silences of a patriarchal discourse on the ideal family. In the framework of such a discourse there is no place for an emotionally charged connection between mother and child that is not already prefigured by a 'moral' law in which a woman's husband has a key place. As Fineman notes, 'the legal story is that a family has a "natural" form based on the sexual affiliation of a man to a woman' (Fineman 1995: 145). This 'sexual family ... simultaneously exists in our social imagination, both as a legal institution and as a cultural ideal with divine credentials. The nuclear family has an assumed "naturalness", venerated in law, institutionalised as the appropriate form of intimacy and secured against defamation or violation by unsanctified alternatives' (Fineman 1995: 150).

This image of the sexual family becomes relevant in the context of new reproductive technologies and surrogacy contracts that make possible the separation of reproduction from the heterosexual relation. It is exactly the naturalness and normality of heterosexual reproduction that people refer to when they argue against the use of reproductive technologies by single women. The second argument is related to the question of acceptability of deliberately creating children who will not have a father. Having a father is considered as normal and natural as heterosexual reproduction and a heterosexual relationship. In the case of SOS Villages, the blame is not about deliberately creating children but about deliberately creating families that do not have a father and hence are *incomplete*. These families are judged this way for two reasons. On the one hand, there is the 'lack of male partner' for the women and on the other, the 'lack of a father' for the children.

The discourse on the 'missing father' certainly contributes to SOS mothers' feeling that their families are somehow not 'normal'. I was able to observe this from the way in which they spoke about different problems related to their family life. They very often used the sentence: 'but this is the same in normal families too'. What surprised me was that the women internalised the discourse about the 'missing father' to such an extent that in some cases they felt guilty and responsible for this 'lack', as if they were to blame for this situation.

The 'missing father' discourse shows clearly the effects of confusing the desirable situation (it is good for the children to have two parents) with the real situation (these children were abandoned by both parents and were raised in institutions where they had neither mother nor father; in the SOS Village they have at least a mother). Even though originally the children raised in the SOS families were born to a 'complete biological family' (meaning that they were born from a heterosexual couple who, in many cases, were either married or cohabiting) for various reasons these families either split up or the biological parents were not able to fulfil their parental responsibilities.[9] Therefore the children ended up in institutions. Thus, it is clear that what is claimed to be the 'normal' structure of a family does not necessarily on its own guarantee the proper functioning of the family.

In many cases the SOS mothers connected the lack of the father with the fact that they are raising these children alone, i.e. that they do not have a male partner with whom they live. Basically, they connect the lack of the father with the lack of a 'husband'. They have to legitimise the fact that they are raising children not only for others, but also for themselves. The fact that most of the mothers make great efforts to supplement the 'missing father' by involving their own family members in the life of their SOS family shows that they somehow feel responsible for this lack and try to correct it. This attitude has been observed by other authors writing about mothers who deliberately decided to become single mothers by giving birth to their children through assisted reproduction or by adoption (Coontz 1992; Bock 2000; Hertz 2002: 26; Jones 2003: 433). From this, I suggest that the ideal image of the family with men and women and their (if possible) biological children is not only a dominant discourse 'out there' but is internalised during socialisation and works through people's unconscious, which is why it has a strong effect on their lives. This explains why the image of the 'ideal' family has a powerful effect on people even in countries where the law and the general public accept, as legitimate, alternative family forms.

It can be concluded that 'the lack of a partner' and 'the lack of a father' problems are internalised by the mothers. They are compelled to legitimise for themselves and for others the fact that their maternal abilities are not linked to their sexual life and that they are also able to play the roles that are generally associated with a male parent. I argue that the discourse on the 'incomplete family' refers to only one missing person in the SOS families: it is neither the sexual partner of a woman, nor a father to the children, but rather a 'man' as the head of the family.

Raising the Children of 'Others'

When analysing what family means for these mothers, we cannot keep the domains of 'the biological' and 'the social' intact, since the distinction between these two aspects is not clear-cut. We can see that once a woman decides to become a foster-mother she often involves her family, who actually support her in raising her foster-children. Many of the foster-mothers try to integrate the foster-children into their own families. The parents of the foster-mother may act as grandparents to the children, while the sisters and brothers of the foster-mother often take the role of the uncle or aunt. Through the affiliation between foster-mother and her children, the children become part of the foster-mother's family of belonging. This process is similar in a way to the process of 'kinning' described by Howell (2001: 208) in the case of adoption, but in some other aspects differs from it. It differs because in the majority of cases the foster-children cannot be adopted by their foster-mothers, so they will never belong formally to her family; for example, they will not transmit the family name, and so on. Yet, in some cases, in everyday life practice, 'grandparents', 'uncles' and 'aunts', the foster-mother and the children act and perceive themselves as a family.[10]

As I have pointed out in the previous section, Hungarians value children highly. However, their attitude towards the SOS mothers' activity suggests that it is not children in general who are valued but only one's own offspring. If this were not the case, the SOS mothers who offer permanent care for children who are 'deprived' of their own families would be appreciated. However, the day-to-day experience of the mothers reveals a different attitude. They claim that many people, and especially men, cannot understand why someone would raise children who are not their own. In the words of one SOS mother:

> It is not the child in itself that is the value, but one's own child. I can see this in my own family: my father is so child-oriented and he loves us so much, but when we grew up and my mother said that we should take a child from the orphanage, he did not even want to listen to her. All the men have the same attitude to this: that another person's child, no way; they say: 'If I could raise my children, other people should do the same; if they decided to have a child, they should also raise it.' (SOS mother)

The higher value of biological ties in comparison with social ties is present not only at the level of social attitude but also at the normative level. The Parliamentary Act on Child Protection, by emphasising the importance of biological ties, reinforces the already existing hierarchisation of biological and social family relations.[11] The SOS organisation's ideology also encourages and contributes to establishing and maintaining the connection between children and their biological parents.[12]

The SOS mothers' experience of being a foster-parent convinced me that it is not easy to be a social parent in an environment where only the biological family ties are the ones that are highly valued. The interviews revealed that the issue of social support is very important for the mothers. Although they receive this support from their family members, they are still concerned with the fact that their work is not accepted and valued by the wider society. They emphasised that, while in Hungary their work is not appreciated by many people, in 'Western' European countries the SOS mothers are respected and their work is highly valued. They told me that, unlike in Hungary, in other countries there is a totally different attitude towards raising children who are not your own:

> In Hungary, even if one adopts a child he or she tries to find one that resembles him or her. In the Netherlands, for example, it is very common for people to raise other children beside their own or, after they have raised their own, to take care of others who for some reason don't have their own family. And, as different as these children may be, for them they are valuable. This is because in that society raising and taking care of children who are not your own are valued by the society, not like here. (SOS mother)

One SOS mother pointed out that in Hungary many people would say there was only one motivation for raising another's children: an economic one.[13] There is, indeed, an unfortunate history of foster-care in Hungary, since it was once a widespread practice to take children from institutions and to use them for work on family farms. The same happened to children of poor families from large cities who were 'given away' to foster-parents in the villages. Hungarian novels, biographies and poems portray the sad stories of such children. With this tradition behind them, the foster mothers try hard to convince people that money is not the reason for choosing to become SOS mothers. Their reaction clearly shows that, in the social context in which they are living, to be paid for being a 'mother' is condemned. This attitude implies that a woman can be a good 'mother' only if her mothering fulfils her 'maternal instinct'.

The fact that the women working in the SOS Children's Village are named 'mothers' has its own significance. If the name of their 'occupation' were, for example, permanent caregiver, it is unlikely that their work would be condemned to the same extent. Women work for a long time as professional caregivers and also get paid for it, but people do not find this provocative in the same way. The name of the professional 'mother' evokes the following problem: if some women get money for doing the 'job' of mothering, would other women go on being 'normal' mothers and continue to consider mothering their duty? Or would they rethink their rights and needs? What appears to be offensive for many Hungarian people is that motherhood may have 'escaped' from the framework of the heterosexual relationship legalised by marriage and that it has become a legally accepted profession and a source of income for some women.

An Imaginary Line of Demarcation: SOS Mothers With or Without Their Own Children

Based on the SOS mothers' narratives one can notice a division between them. I could see after a while that the mothers were divided into two groups, but it took me some time to figure out the lines along which the boundaries of exclusion and inclusion were constructed in this community. Although the mothers were usually friendly with each other, I found that none of the mothers had a close relationship with a mother from the 'other' group. I realised that this division had a particular significance for the women and came to understand that the line of demarcation between the women coincided with whether they had a child of their own or not.

The background of having or not having their own biological children influences the way in which SOS mothers construct and define their understanding of motherhood. Those women who have no children of their own told me that they love the children they are raising, as they would love their own. However, they are often told that their feelings are not what a 'real' mother, that is, a biological mother, feels:

> I think that even a foster-child can be loved in the same way as one's own. But I don't have my own child. I was always told – by schoolmates, friends – that it is different to have one's own children. I asked why it is different. They said, it is different, believe us, it is different. We couldn't agree because I kept saying that the child becomes my own since I take care of it, I am at his or her bedside if she or he is ill, I am there when there are problems, and this is what matters. They say that it is the nine months, the giving birth that makes it different. (SOS mother)

This SOS mother did not want to admit that being a biological mother is a different experience from being a social one. Our discussion revealed that the reason for her insistence on the denial of the difference was not connected with her inability to be aware of the difference itself, but was related to a broader attitude in relation to differences, that is, that difference always implies a hierarchy. Knowing the social context in which this discussion took place, it is not difficult to see that once the difference is admitted, one of the two kinds of motherhood would be assigned a lower status and this would not be biological motherhood. When I suggested to her that a difference would not necessarily imply a hierarchy of value, thus pointing out that the difference between biological and social motherhood should not mean that one is more valuable than the other, she told me that this somehow had never occurred to her. As she said at the end of our discussion, she found this 'new' insight empowering and she thought it would help her to come to terms with the problem.

Those women who have their own biological children 'admitted' that they love their own children more and emphasised the importance of biological ties. One of the mothers, for example, thinks that a foster-mother has to be very aware of the limits of her parenting:

> I would lie if I affirmed that I don't love my own children more. Blood is thicker than water ('a vér nem válik vizzé') I always say that.[14] A lot depends on blood relations and I told M. [her foster-child] as well, if I slapped you that would be totally different, you would never forget it, it would be very humiliating, especially at this age; if your mom slapped you, you would forget all about it in a week's time. These children can condemn their own parents, but I know that I cannot say a single negative word about them; I can scold my own parents, my own children, but nobody else can do it; and I know this very well, that is how it works. (SOS mother)

It is not easy for any of the SOS mothers to define their identity and to position themselves within many, often contradictory, discourses. However, I found that for those women who are both biological and social mothers, it is a more difficult task. While those women who are not biological mothers emphasise responsibility as a determining feature of being a good parent, those who have their own children emphasised the importance of biological ties. Nevertheless, they find themselves in a difficult position. On the one hand, they affirm that there is something important in the biological act of giving birth that also influences one's parenting. On the other hand, their actual job requires them to be a good parent for their foster-children. But how can they be a 'good parent' of a foster-child if they are convinced that one's parenting abilities are determined by the act of birth?

This uncertainty of SOS mothers in defining their position in the discourse about the biological and social aspects of motherhood can be observed in their narratives. There are several levels that can be traced in our discussion. First of all, every biological mother 'confessed' that she loved her own children more and that the relationship with them is 'special'. They also seemed to believe that giving birth is the determining factor of being a 'true' parent. However, when talking about their foster-children's biological mother, one SOS mother said with genuine surprise and wonder:

> If she was a 'real' mother, if she had any maternal feelings, she would never do this [abandon her children]. There was not even a flash in her eyes or any kind of emotion on her face, no nothing. She just sat there [when once she visited her children in the SOS village]. She cannot be a real mother. (SOS mother)

We can see the contextuality of emphasising one or the other element of motherhood – biological connection or responsibility – as it would be 'a partisan act to take one or the other element as indicative and definitive of kinship' (Edwards, this volume). Those mothers who claim that 'giving birth' is what makes a woman a 'real' mother find themselves in a difficult position when they have to explain the basis of their foster-parenthood. If they believe that true parenthood is determined by biology and that giving birth is what constitutes real motherhood, how do so many 'real' mothers end up abandoning their children?

The 'presence' of a birth mother is discomfiting for many foster-mothers. In a society 'where legal rights might be lost, but the blood relationship cannot be lost' (Schneider 1968: 24) and where the legal system prioritises biological ties over social ones, the existence of a birth mother is a constant reminder to the foster-mothers that their tie to their children may not be such an enduring tie as the ties of blood. This could be one of the reasons why some SOS mothers have difficulties in accepting biological mothers.

But what does a biological tie mean for these women? When we try to find an answer to this question we have to take into consideration that in the context of this fieldwork it was not assumed that the genetic and biological aspects of motherhood could be separated. For these women, giving birth to their own child meant also giving birth to a child who is genetically connected to them. It is evident that some of the mothers strongly emphasised pregnancy and giving birth as the features of biological parenthood, but this happened because they were not speaking about parenthood in general, but about motherhood specifically. Interestingly, these women mentioned the genetic connection when they discussed general attitudes towards raising their own or other people's children, or when they pointed out that it is more important for men to have their own children. While it might happen that biological fathers would emphasise that genes are transmitted to their children when defining what it means for them to have their own child, the mothers emphasised what is specific in being a biological mother: and this specificity is not sharing genes but pregnancy and birth. However, this does not mean that sharing genes is not important for them. What can be concluded is that based on the women's narratives, for them a biological tie means both notions of sharing genes and other forms of biological bonding, such as giving birth, and it is impossible to differentiate between the two.

Ultimately, the mothers' narratives lead us to debates on the determining features of parenthood and to questions such as what makes someone a real mother or what it means to have your own child.[15] Is the real mother the one who gave birth to the child, or the one whom the child resembles, or is it perhaps the one who takes responsibility for raising the child? Is there only one real mother? A monistic account of parenthood, based on the principle that one and only one thing – genes, gestation or intention – can be the basis of parenthood cannot account for all categories of motherhood.[16] Parenthood is always embedded in a context, and real-life situations have a great influence on who is and who is not a real parent. Only a pluralist account of parenthood can do justice to this contextual embeddedness of meanings and interpretations of parenthood and relatedness. According to such an account, depending on the context, any of the above-mentioned factors – genetics, biology, care and responsibility – can constitute the basis for parenthood (Bayne and Kolers 2003b).

Conclusion

Due to the specifics of their situation, SOS foster-mothers have to interpret and reinterpret the cultural meanings linked to motherhood in order to define their own identity. As noted above, they have to construct, define and legitimise their identity as single women and single mothers within the framework of an institution which is different from marriage. At the same time, they interpret their mothering not (just) as an innate duty, but as an acquired skill and a profession.

One of the most interesting features of the foster-mothers' narratives is the controversial schism in women's perception of biological and social motherhood, along with their unawareness of it. The schism is clearly based on the underlying dualistic nature of the discourse on motherhood (as well as any other existent discourse) and the lack of awareness of the implications such dualism creates. First, these women cannot accept this duality because the rigid exclusion and hierarchisation of one concept over another is inherent in our 'dualistic' society. Secondly, to accept that the difference of the biological motherhood experience does not imply more value than social mothering is discouraged by the hierarchisation of values. Thirdly, the ambiguity is located in the implicit presence of an 'other' mother in the life of their children. Foster-motherhood constitutes therefore a space where the experience of identity and connection and the experience of contingency and separation converge powerfully providing in this way compelling insights that connect with current debates about biological and social aspects of relatedness.

The SOS foster mothers' narratives of motherhood, family and relatedness show us that different ways of imagining kin connections are readily mobilised by these mothers. Their narratives reveal that intention and agency as well as non-intention and the lack of agency are both present in the making, breaking and sustaining of intimate social relations, highlight the indeterminacy of 'biological facts' and disclose diverse strategies of making kinship. Kinship from this perspective is made up of a number of heterogeneous elements, and the context and intention determines which of them will be deployed and put to the fore in a particular instance.

Analysing the professional foster-mother's experience on motherhood and family in Hungary, we can see that the dominant discourses about family, parenthood, relatedness and gender identity are not only cognitive 'constructions' 'out there', but deeply affect the lives of those who occupy marginal positions in connection with these dominant norms. Making these marginal experiences visible could represent a first step for recognition and support for diverse family arrangements in everyday life, in public policy and in law and could contribute to the rethinking of some of our ideas on relatedness.

Notes

I wish to express my gratitude to Judit Sándor for suggesting the SOS Village to me as a good site for research about motherhood. The fieldwork was carried out with the support of a Central European University Gender Department Small Grant programme. The article was further developed in the framework of the 'Public Understanding of Genetics' (PUG) project. I would like to thank all PUG colleagues for the interesting exchange of ideas on new ways of looking at kinship, and the editors of this book for their useful and indeed constructive comments on earlier drafts of this chapter. Last but not least, special thanks to the SOS mothers from the SOS Village of Kecskemét; without their willingness to share with me their experiences of being a foster-mother this chapter could not have been written.

1. For more information about this organisation see the web page http://www.sos-childrensvillages.org/, accessed on 14 October 2005.
2. Kecskemét is a city located 85 km from Hungary's capital, Budapest. There are three SOS Children's Villages in Hungary. The first village was set up in 1986, and that in Kecskemét in 1988. This latter SOS Children's Village is located in a residential area of the city and consists of twelve family houses, a community house and the house of the village directors. Each of the eleven SOS mothers who were working in the village during my fieldwork had her 'own' house, where she raised four to seven children.
3. In line with a Foucauldian understanding, I define discourse not only as text (language), but also as social practice.
4. For more information see World Value Survey, Hungary.
5. See ibid.
6. These statements are based on the data of the Census of the Hungarian Central Statistical Office, 2001.
7. The number of children and young adults placed in children's homes and foster-care in 2003 was 21,122. See *Yearbook of Welfare Statistics* (2004) p. 51.
8. See Hungarian Act No. XXXI of 1997 on Child Protection.
9. It is also interesting to note that the majority of those SOS mothers who have their own biological children gave birth to their children in the framework of marriage and a 'normal' family. But all of them got divorced and ended up raising their own children alone.
10. This is not happening, however, in every case. There are foster-mothers who get involved more in raising the children, while others keep more of a distance. My point here is that where there is an intention to integrate these children in the mothers' family this can be achieved.
11. A similar tendency has been noted in the case of Norwegian legislation and public discourse (Howell 2001; Melhuus 2003; Melhuus and Howell, this volume).

12. This was not always the case. The organisation changed its policy regarding the relationship with the biological mother based on the children's right to know their families (Jeddi 2003).
13. The economic reason for taking children into foster-care is mentioned by Cadoret in her ethnography on foster-parenthood in the region of Morvan, France (Cadoret 1995: 83–86).
14. '*A vér nem válik vízzé*': the literal translation into English is 'the blood will never become water'.
15. See more on the topic of 'having one's own child' in Melhuus (2007) and Bestard (this volume).
16. For a philosophical account of parenthood see, for example, Bayne and Kolers (2003a).

CHAPTER 9

Adoption and Assisted Conception:
One Universe of Unnatural Procreation.
An Examination of Norwegian Legislation

Marit Melhuus and Signe Howell

On Thursday, 14 October 2004, one of Norway's major tabloid newspapers ran the following headline: 'King Haakon was not [King] Olav's father?' The subtext reads: 'In his new book on the monarchy, biographer Tor Bomann-Larsen suggests that Sir Francis Laking, the king's personal doctor, is King Olav's biological father.'[1] The following day, several newspapers ran a follow-up and this news item even merited international attention. The *Daily Mirror* (UK) had the following headline: 'Was a King of Norway really made in England?' *Timesonline* ran an article titled 'The "British" royals of Norway'.[2] The opening sentence reads: 'A British baronet secretly sired the late King of Norway using a primitive form of artificial insemination, according to a new biography that casts doubt on the Norwegian royal bloodline.'

This is an unusual story. It deals with sperm donation and artificial insemination carried out in 1902, and draws attention to the possible illegitimate status of the late king and, by implication, that of the present king and crown prince. The event took place before Norway obtained its independence from Sweden and became a sovereign state in 1905. The event also predates the decision of the young Norwegian state to opt for a constitutional monarchy (rather than a republic) and its choice of Prince Carl of Denmark to become King Haakon VII of Norway. Prince Carl was married to his cousin Princess Maud, the daughter of King Edward VII and granddaughter of Queen Victoria. Maud and Carl had been childless for six years when their son Alexander Edward Christian Fredrik was born. This was the boy who later became King Olav V of Norway. It is the authenticity of his bloodline that is being questioned by the allegation of conception by donor sperm. Thus, the story has the ingredients of a scandal: insinuating that the Norwegian royal family was compromised before it became installed. The story challenges the royal imperative of impeccable descent lines predicated upon biological connectedness and patriarchy, and introduces the uncertainty of paternity.

Bomann-Larsen (2004) builds his case on circumstantial evidence. Hence he has no direct proof of what he suggests, although his arguments, not least the photographic evidence, appear convincing.[3] However, of one thing he is sure: Princess Maud did give birth to a son. He was not adopted. Thus, the author refutes the rumour, which circulated at the time that the child was adopted, a rumour that the Nazis nurtured during the occupation of Norway during the Second World War in order to slander King Haakon, who headed the Norwegian government in exile in London and was the symbol of Norwegian resistance. If headlines and media debates are anything to go by, the news was received as sensational. Nevertheless, perhaps the most sensational aspect of this piece of information – at least in the context of this chapter – is that the possible conception by donor sperm of the former king of Norway ultimately has not made a difference to the status of the royal family. The Norwegian public does not seem to be affected in their high opinion of the monarchy, or in their opinion of King Olav.[4] After the first flurry of excitement, the possible doubt about the purity of the royal descent line did not have serious consequences for the current royal family, let alone create a constitutional crisis. In light of our own research on kinship in Norway, we find it surprising that this news did not evoke strong moral or emotional reactions among the public at large, as it goes against an accepted understanding of succession. At first sight, it also runs counter to our findings that there is an increasing preoccupation with biology, not least with biogenetic origins in matters of personal identity, and that public discourses on kinship are characterised by an increasing tendency to 'biologise' identities and kin relatedness (e.g. Howell 2001, 2003; Howell and Melhuus 2001; Melhuus 2007). The incident demonstrates the opposite; namely a willingness to grant kin-status as a result of social intimacy. Thus, we let this incident stand as a marker for the complexity of values and meanings tied to the significance of family relations and biological relations in contemporary Norway.

Although this chapter will not deal with kings, or royal families and their descent lines, this news item draws attention to issues that we shall address: values concerning the meaning of family formation and kin relatedness and the tension between social and biological forms of belonging. By focusing on 'unnatural' forms of procreation, assisted conception and adoption, we argue that values about what is natural and normal are thrown into sharp relief. The story of the king's biological origins lends a historical dimension to involuntary childlessness and the solutions that those concerned resorted to. It marks the continuity of this problem and draws attention to the relatively recent developments in new reproductive technologies (NRT). Thus, we are also alerted to some fundamental changes in sociocultural values over the past hundred years with regard to the meaning of belonging and kinship. In effect, we suggest that these 'unnatural' forms of procreation are in the process of being naturalised. This process is reflected in changes in legislation throughout the century.

Assisted Procreation: Adoption and Assisted Conception

In what follows, we assume that assisted conception (including new reproductive technologies and artificial insemination by donor – AID) and adoption are social phenomena that belong to the same order and should therefore be examined together as mutually implicated forms of assisted procreation. Despite their intrinsic link, however, adoption and assisted conception have rarely been seen in conjunction by anthropologists or other social scientists. Our suggestion is that by examining them in parallel, exploring their continuities as well as discontinuities, the understanding of each practice is enhanced (see also Howell and Melhuus 2007). Moreover, the approach contributes to a new understanding of kinship, both as a theoretical concept and a social category, something that is both empirically and analytically justified.

We argue that there has been an increasing biologisation of discourses about identity and personhood in Norway over the past few years. This is occurring in a cultural climate that has come to celebrate the values of autonomy and self-realisation: an ideology that is reflected in legal provisions and policy debates (we shall return to this). Through endless articles and TV programmes dealing with issues related to family, children, involuntary childlessness and transnational adoption, the media demonstrate a general preoccupation with the biological foundation of kinship, the case of King Olav's dubious conception being but one example. This convergence of biology and individual autonomy is made possible through an identity discourse that subsumes and collapses specific notions of biogenetic relatedness and notions of rights. The gist of the argument is as follows: To know your biological origin is tantamount to knowing who you are, and this knowledge is today presented as a right. The forcefulness of this argumentation has come to permeate public discourses to such a degree that to argue otherwise is considered not only irrational but virtually unethical.[5]

Within the Norwegian procreative universe – which includes NRT and transnational adoption – it is possible to discern a preoccupation with the constituting significance of biogenetics. Most significantly this has to do with the nature/nurture configuration and the shifting articulations of the values placed on one at the expense of the other. However, as practices, they represent two different trends: one that privileges the biological over the social (NRT) and the other that privileges, albeit somewhat uneasily, the social over the biological (adoption). As sociocultural trends they underlie a series of potentially contentious issues. Both involve, *inter alia*, questions of secrecy and anonymity, inheritance, marriage, socialisation, authenticity and belonging. While these issues are particularly in evidence in contemporary Norway, our perusal of historical documents and legislative processes demonstrates that they have been of concern since the beginning of the twentieth century.

To explore the meanings and practices generated by gamete donation and adoption is fruitful because these phenomena directly and indirectly challenge the biogenetic basis of kin relatedness. This is all the more compelling since the people directly concerned, i.e. those opting for either gamete donation or adoption, tend to stress the relational quality of the parent-child relationship rather than the biogenetic one (Melhuus 2007).

Legislating and Legislation

In line with Foucault (1991) and Rose (1999), we see law as a primary technology of government, and family forms can be said to be crafted through laws (Sterett 2002: 223; Howell 2006). However, the law regulating assisted conception (and its subsequent revisions) can also be seen as an attempt on the part of government to keep pace with the technological changes within reproductive medicine. We shall show how, in contemporary Norway, the laws pertaining to adoption and assisted conception are in some ways imbricated, despite the fact that these laws spring out of different contexts of expertise and appeared at different historical times (see below). Whereas adoption laws belong to the corpus of laws dealing with children and the family passed during the first decade of the twentieth century, the laws on assisted conception fall under biotechnology and medicine, which are much more recent.

In the following, we explore the kinds of attitudes towards adoption and NRT by examining the relevant legal frameworks, the codification of laws and the concomitant legislative processes. Laws are significant because they both reflect dominant social concerns and values and are normative, in the sense that they seek to regulate and/or improve current practices. Because laws are cumulative, changes in the cultural climate are easy to trace. Furthermore, because laws are explicit and unequivocal in their formulations, it is possible to identify the moral principles that are evoked and challenged. Points of contention are invariably expressed in White Papers and parliamentary debates surrounding legal codification of policy decisions. Hence, legislative processes are instructive in that they reveal significant strands of public understanding, in this case, of biogenetic relatedness.

This approach allows us to identify those areas where thinking about adoption and assisted conception converge. A closer examination of the legislation and legislative processes concerning adoption and assisted conception serves to highlight shifting positions with regard to the significance of biogenetic and social bonds (see also Dalton 2000; Borneman 2001; Kahn 2002). Thus, laws provide an important window through which one may view contemporary values.

It is important to keep in mind that government in Norway is based on the principles of the welfare state. Trägårdh argues that 'the central organising principle of the Nordic welfare state ... is the *alliance* between the state and the individual' (Trågårdh 1997: 253; italics in original). If this contention is correct, it would follow that notions of (individual) rights find fertile ground. Moreover, the image of the state is one of a potential instrument of reform rather than repression (Sørensen and Stråth 1997: 7). State interference in private and personal matters is the rule rather than the exception.[6] The Norwegian state operates according to an ideology that increasingly has supported public involvement in family life in general and in adoption and assisted conception in particular. Laws are made on behalf of society, and society is to a certain extent perceived as coterminous with the state. Thus, underpinning legislative processes – almost as a precondition – is a fundamental attitude based on an abstract trust between government and the people. In matters related to adoption and assisted conception, state intervention has been deemed necessary and there has been an explicit will to govern (Melhuus 2005a; Howell 2006). Examining the changing and concurrent legislation within adoption and assisted conception brings this out clearly.

In the case of the Norwegian laws concerning adoption and assisted conception, the sociocultural elements involved not only go to the core of the liberal state and its dilemma of individual freedom versus state control, but also strike at the premises for life and significant relationships. Here we have in mind the status of the embryo, the status of the child, the question of individual rights and the significance attributed to biogenetic bonds, as well as questions related to marriage, paternity and maternity. The meanings attached to these categories have undergone some subtle, and yet eventually, fundamental transformations. That important changes have taken place is exemplified by the case mentioned in the introduction of the late King Olav. No matter what the source of his conception was, the rule of *pater est quem nuptiae demonstrant* (marriage defines who the father is) automatically made the young prince the legal son of the future King Haakon, because he was married to Maud, the prince's mother and future queen. According to Norwegian legal thinking, until very recently, marriage was the relationship that defined legitimacy. As Cadoret (this volume) points out, this was the case in general for western societies. Marriage was the institution that ensured filiation, providing the framework for accepted procreation and sexuality. Today, this is no longer the case. In Norway, recent laws recognise paternity as based primarily on biogenetic relatedness ascertained through DNA tests, thus directly undermining the rule of *pater est*.[7] Biological paternity is now regarded as paramount in the sense that a man may unilaterally request a DNA test in order to ascertain the paternity of a child, regardless of the marital status of the mother of the child.[8] This is only one of many indicators that underpin a tendency to give increasing significance to the relationship mother-child/father-child at the expense of the family as a social unit. The very prohibition of egg donation in Norway serves to uphold certainty about who the mother is, as no distinction may be made between biogenetic mother and birth mother (Melhuus 2003). This is further exemplified by changes in the naming laws. These have shifted from following descent with a patrilineal tendency, to cognatic or matrilineal (see below).

At the same time, legal marriage has lost its central position as more and more couples choose cohabitation as a preferred basis for creating a family. This has meant that the distinction between legitimate and illegitimate children has disappeared (Melhuus 2001; see also Teichman 1982) and that the notion of the 'illegitimate child' no longer exists as a meaningful category in Norway. In many ways, the disappearance of the illegitimate child sums up a series of sociocultural changes that have occurred in Norwegian society with regard to sexuality, gender relations and family constitution. In fact, we suggest that this loss of meaning of illegitimacy entails the idea that all children are morally equal and is thus a prerequisite for the development of the rights of the child. It is also a significant contributing factor to the rapid acceptance of new forms of assisted procreation – both transnational adoption and new reproductive technologies.

The notions of the best interest of the child and child rights have penetrated the social order to such a degree that from a formal point of view the child is seen as an individual in its own right, irrespective of the relationships it embodies. Yet underpinning all these changes is a notion that blood is, after all, thicker than water. The sense of this notion has, however, changed. Whereas blood relations earlier were taken to be coterminous with the legally constituted family, today in Norway 'blood' has become limited to biogenetic relations and denotes 'origin' and 'identity', irrespective of the social relations involved.

Adoption: 1917–1956

By itself, adoption is necessarily a challenge to any form of kinship system that either bases itself ontologically upon biogenetic connectedness or that, minimally, uses such connectedness to constitute a systematic understanding of relatedness. Since adoption breaks with theories of reproduction that are ontologically grounded in biogenetics, local explanations and practices of adoption become interesting, in particular with regard to dilemmas that are thought to arise. Viewed in conjunction with assisted conception, and more specifically those involving gamete donation, these dilemmas become all the more apparent.

Over the recent past there has been, in Norway, a rapid increase in the practice of adopting children from overseas. This began in the late 1960s, when couples began to adopt children from Korea and Vietnam. Since that time, Norwegians have been adopting children from more than twenty countries. Thus, in contrast to Hungary (Demény, this volume) Norwegians are not reluctant to raise children who are not (biogenetically) 'their own'. On the contrary, the demand for transnationally adopted children is steadily increasing. The move to adopt transnationally coincided with the reduction of Norwegian-born babies made available for adoption in Norway. The reasons for this are many but, most importantly, it has to do with fundamental changes in attitudes to sexuality, motherhood and marriage. Contraception and abortion became generally available.[9] Moreover, the stigma attached to being an unwed mother (as it was called then) disappeared.

Although adoption and fostering practices were well established in Norway, there was no legal apparatus that regulated adoption until the first Norwegian Adoption Law, entitled 'To forge a link', was passed in 1917.[10] It was nine years ahead of the first English legislation (Ingvaldsen 1996) and amongst the first in Europe. The main purpose of the 1917 law was to meet a need arising out of involuntary childlessness of well-situated couples, which was stated as 'a desire to see their name and family continue'. At the same time, it was also understood, but not much elaborated, that adoption should benefit the child as well. Paragraph 8, for example, states that '[permission to adopt] must not be given unless there is good reason to assume that it will serve the interest of the child'. At the time, children put up for adoption were mainly illegitimate children whose prospects otherwise, especially in the rapidly growing urban areas, were pretty grim (Ingvaldsen 1996: 10). Most commentators, however, agree that the 1917 act catered primarily for the needs of the adoptive parents and their biological kin.

The 1917 act came in the aftermath of more than two decades of codifications of a series of laws that sought to protect weaker groups in Norwegian society. A concern for the plight of illegitimate children resulted in a series of Children's Acts at the beginning of the twentieth century, the so-called Castberg Children's Acts, named after the politician responsible for formulating them (see also Teichman 1982: 165–67). These acts became a model for subsequent acts in other European countries and were acclaimed for their liberal attitudes. Of the six separate acts that made up the Children's Act, four were concerned with children born outside wedlock. Much of the debate surrounding these laws was concerned with the right of a child born outside of marriage to bear the name of the progenitor and to inherit from him (assuming of course that his identity was known, which was often the case). The opponents feared that the name and inheritance rights would undermine marriage and family life. Others objected to the public interference in private life that this law was seen to represent. In 1915 one commentator stated: 'When the state decides about the most intimate aspects of the most intimate relations, then soon our home will no longer be our own but the state's' (Ingvaldsen 1996:10). Thus, the tension between private matters and public interest was already being voiced.

Until the amendment in 1979 of the Naming Law of 1964, surnames in Norway followed the agnatic principle whereby a legally married wife and the children of the marriage automatically took the husband and father's surname.[11] Surnames, of course, are par excellence about relatedness and relational identity, as also Cadoret's (this volume) example about homoparental families in France indicates. Particular names denote not just the parent-child relationship, but also the wider kin, both lineally and laterally. The kin name denotes belonging, with all the moral connotations that this involves. The question of the adopted child's name was, not surprisingly, problematic. The 1917 law clearly reflects a strong belief in the importance of a biological basis for kin ties that are reckoned in the agnatic line. By conferring his surname on a child, a man's paternal status is confirmed. Indeed, the right granted to adoptees to revert to the surname of their biological father reflects this. In practice most adoptees took their adoptive father's surname, but the right to revert was considered sufficiently important for it to be safe-guarded.

An implicit understanding about the meaning of kinship upholds the biological connection as primary (Ingvaldsen 1996: 17, Howell 2006). Thus, the legal links of adopted children to their biological parents were not severed. They kept all rights to equal inheritance from them. By extension, the biological parents had rights of inheritance from the child they had given up for adoption, and some rights to financial support. By the same token, the law gave priority to biological children if there were any, and adopted children could only inherit a small portion of their adoptive parents' property. To equate an adopted child with a biological one was not even debated in the preamble to the 1917 act. But the responsibility for the adoptee's upkeep was passed to its adoptive parents. At the same time, the adoptive parents did not have rights of inheritance or rights to maintenance from their adopted child. Property was to be kept within the bloodline. Blood was clearly perceived as thicker than water in the eyes of the law. In 1923 a minor amendment to the 1917 Adoption Law was passed that removed an adoptee's automatic right to revert to his or her original name, making the break with biological relatives complete. If the adoptee desired to use that name, he or she had to apply for permission.

The preoccupation with the rights of parents is manifest in the amendment of 1935 when two kinds of adoption were made legal, the so-called weak adoption, whereby the adoptive parents might revoke the relationship if the child was 'unsatisfactory' (Ingvaldsen 1996: 53), and strong adoption, whereby revocation was made impossible and all legal ties with the biological family were severed. This decision must be viewed in relation to debates about eugenics and 'racial hygiene' that were prevalent in Norway during the first half of the twentieth century, debates and concomitant practices that have also had implications for the formulation of legislation regarding assisted conception, albeit from a totally different perspective (see below). There was a strong concern with containing bad genes and encouraging good ones, and poverty was to some extent linked to the idea of bad genes (Roll-Hansen and Broberg 1996). Many adoptive parents were on the lookout for the manifestation of bad genes in an adopted child, and the weak version of the adoption law was meant to provide a let-out for adoptive parents. A revised adoption law was passed in 1944 that enabled the revocation of an adoption if it was discovered that the child was chronically ill or handicapped (Ingvaldsen 1996: 20). Such 'deficiencies' had to date back prior to the time of adoption, and submission to revoke had to be made within five years of the adoption itself. The 1948 amendment opened the way for adoption even if a couple had biological children, so long as they were deemed good parents. Moreover, the duty to support biological parents was repealed. This amendment both reflected a backward glance (the best interest of the parents) and anticipated a forward one (the best interest of the child). The next amendment came in 1956 when strong adoption became the only type allowed – a practice that by this time had become the norm.

Although the first adoption laws arose in the wake of a concern for the plight of illegitimate children, their purpose was to meet the needs of well-situated, involuntary childless couples. The laws explicitly privileged a biological basis for kin ties, and this was reflected in the debates about surname and inheritance rights. This was most acutely articulated through the special rights to *odel*, which gives a male in the direct line (the eldest son) the right to inherit or re-appropriate the family farm. The right to *odel* or *odelsrett* was a descent right of the primogenitor, not a family right, stressing both the significance of blood ties and the agnatic line. The Norwegian Law of *Odel* was not changed until 1974, when both biological daughters and adoptees could claim the right, i.e. the oldest child, irrespective of sex and biogenetic tie to the parents. The gradual shift in the adoption laws reflects an overall change in attitudes to family and children. With the 1956 amendment, the notion of the best interest of the child gains ground.

During the early post-war period the social and natural aspects of adoption became emphasised. The term 'social parents' was introduced for the first time in the 1956 amendments, marking an acceptance of the overriding significance of environmental factors in bringing up children. At this time the state took upon itself a more active role in family politics and child-care. To find suitable parents for unwanted children became a public responsibility.

Assisted Conception: 1950–2003

At about the same time as the Adoption Law was being amended in 1956, the earliest attempts were made to regulate assisted conception, when there was a Nordic effort to coordinate legislation. In 1950 the Norwegian government appointed a committee to review questions related to artificial insemination by donor (AID). It was known that artificial insemination was being practised (Løvset 1951) and the committee was asked to evaluate the need and conditions for AID as well as the legal status of the child. The committee submitted its report, called 'Innstilling fra Inseminasjonskomitéen', in 1953, the majority suggesting that legislation be passed permitting artificial insemination with anonymous donor sperm. However, no legislation was passed until 1987.[12]

Along with public debates in newspapers and other publications at the time (Løvset 1951; Rønne-Pettersen 1951; Sandemose 1952), this official document is interesting as it reflects the shifting moral ground and values of the time. The committee assumed the rule of *pater est* (thereby resolving the legal status of the child) and took for granted the institution of marriage. In fact, the conjugal relation was seen as the nexus around which other relations gravitated. The debates *pro et contra* AID tended to pivot around the nature – nurture configuration expressed in terms of biology and psychology and the moral connotations these evoke with regard to what is natural, good and right. Keeping in mind that the context for this report coincides with the 1956 amendment to the Adoption Law (repealing the weak form of adoption), it is pertinent to draw out the main framing of the arguments. These centred on the significance of the institution of marriage, the home and love, on the one hand, and women's natural desire to have children and the significance of infertility for masculine identity, on the other. Lying and the introduction of a third party in marriage (through AID) are themes that are reiterated. The most controversial issue, however, was that of the anonymity of the donor, a controversy that reverberates to this day.

Anonymity, as it was understood at the time, implied secrecy. It is therefore interesting to examine the question of anonymity in light of the practice of secrecy with regard to adopted children. No versions of the Norwegian adoption laws specified or encouraged secrecy about the adoptive relationship. In the period preceding and following the 1917 Adoption Act there was full acknowledgement of the non-biological status of the relationship. However, by the 1950s (which is the period when the first attempts to legislate AID were made), it had become common practice to pretend that the adopted child was one's own biological child (Ingvaldsen 1996). The post-war period was characterised by an explanatory shift from the determining significance of biology (nature) to environmental factors (nurture), a shift that can be explained as a reaction to the ideology of racial hygiene and Nazism, as well as the growing significance of psychology. Hence, the practice of pretence and secrecy is somewhat paradoxical, and yet it can be understood in terms of prevalent family values. The 1950s were a time when family and family life were idealised and the model of women as mothers, housewives and homemakers became dominant. Motherhood was the manifestation of successful womanhood. Indeed, psychological literature of the 1950s explained childlessness in women as the result of psychological abnormality (Leira 1996: 133), thus putting enormous pressure on the women concerned. Infertility was a condition to be concealed and many women who failed to produce a child tried in secret to find a child to adopt. Adoption thus became a shameful activity, and the fact of adoption was a well-kept secret even from the adoptees themselves.

In so far as this was the dominant attitude, it is perhaps not surprising that the majority in the committee set to evaluate the possible legislation of AID had few qualms about the use of anonymous donor sperm. At that time, the use of known sperm donors was not even discussed. Donor anonymity would not only hide a man's infertility (a condition that was rarely recognised), but it would also give the wife a possibility of becoming a mother. Moreover, the practice of adoption was used as an argument in favour of legislating for AID. The adoptive parent – adopted child relation (more specifically, the stepfather – stepchild relation) was held up as exemplary of the love one can feel for a child that is not biologically one's own, the implication being that AID will not undermine the love of the father for (t)his child. Rather AID was seen (by those who were for legislating this practice) as strengthening the marriage relation. The reasons for this were varied and tied as much to the importance of being a family as they were to the importance of married women becoming mothers. In fact, the significance of the institution of marriage at the time must not be underestimated. A good home was seen as equivalent to a good marriage, and marriage was considered to be a fundamental principle of society.

For those against AID, having children was not considered a precondition for a happy marriage; the relationship between the spouses was. If the desire for children was very strong, adoption was considered the best alternative. Adoption, it was maintained, ensured that both parents had the same relation to the child (an argument that adoptive parents and the involuntarily childless reiterate today) and 'moreover, a child that is adopted already exists and the spouses feel they can give it better opportunities than it otherwise would have' (Ministry of Justice 1953: 53). Insemination was seen as a violation of a natural process and being capable of having unimaginable consequences; adoption, however, was a better alternative because 'the adopted child's becoming (*tilblivelse*) is natural, just as adoption in itself is both natural and well known ... and it does not violate any biological mechanism' (Ministry of Justice 1953: 55). Thus three prominent arguments related to adoption are disclosed: one has to do with the relation of the parents to the child; the second has to do with what can be termed charitable motives (giving the adopted child a better chance in life); and the third has to do with adoption, after all, being 'natural'.

Perhaps the most important argument against legislation of AID was that AID 'hides the truth and demands secrecy about a series of interdependent human relations ... as well as deviating from the principle of responsibility of biological fatherhood' (Ministry of Justice 1953: 56). This argument was linked to the opinion that legislation would generate a general doubt about origins and that 'the donor child will lack knowledge of its origins and thereby of itself' (Ministry of Justice 1953:

56). Although this identity argument was not very prominent at the time, it is one that has gradually won ground, and is in contemporary Norway the dominant position held: knowledge of biological origin is fundamental to identity. This was confirmed in the Adoption Law of 1986. The important thing to note, however, is that both secrecy (in adoption) and anonymity (in sperm donation) served to uphold the foundational notion of biological relatedness (see also Haimes 1992). These unnatural procreative practices were hidden from the public gaze; only a few selected people were privy to the knowledge. The children were presented as if they were the biological children of the couple concerned. However, with the advent of transnational adoption such pretence was not possible; the children very clearly did not look like their parents. One visible result was an openness about childlessness, and the stigma attached to adoption was largely lifted. However, AID with donor anonymity remained enveloped in silence, and, when the first legislation was passed in 1987, donor anonymity was upheld. The main argument at the time was that rescinding donor anonymity would result in fewer donors (Melhuus 2001, 2003).

The event that finally prompted legislation on assisted conception was the birth of the first *in vitro* fertilised (IVF) child in Norway in 1984. Fertilisation *ex utero* was now a reality, more than thirty years since the first consideration of legislating for AID. The fact that Norwegian doctors had succeeded in producing an IVF baby made evident that new reproductive technologies were developing at a pace that demanded some form of legislation – lest 'matters get out of hand'. Government intervention was deemed appropriate, also by medical practitioners. Moreover, the increasing public awareness of the procedures (not least fuelled by the sensational headlines surrounding IVF) also made infertility and involuntary childlessness a public issue. The political climate was now conducive to legislation (see Melhuus 2005a).

The first law to regulate assisted conception in Norway was passed in 1987. This law was also among the first in the world. The law was revised in 1994 (the Act Relating to the Application of Biotechnology in Medicine), and assisted conception was included in the same law as other biomedical procedures. Revisions were made again in 2003.[13] The most important revision of relevance in this context was that the anonymity clause was revoked, the argument being that to deny a child the right to know its biological origin is to deny it its identity. The actual law regulates assisted conception, research on embryos and cloning, prenatal screening, genetic screening, genetic therapy and pre-implantation diagnostics. The law is one of the most restrictive in Europe. The law permits sperm donation but only with a known donor; the law does not permit donation of ova, stating that fertilised eggs must be returned to the woman from whom the egg cells were removed (paragraph 2–15). However, an earlier prohibition of the combination of IVF with donor sperm was removed and permission to store egg cells granted. Assisted conception is only open to heterosexual couples. Research on embryos is not permitted. Prenatal screening is only permitted in exceptional cases; genetic therapy on the fetus and on embryos is prohibited, as is genetic therapy that may cause genetic changes to sex cells.

Two more points relevant for our argument must be added: (1) The law states that the couple should be informed about the medical and legal implications of treatment, and they must also be informed about adoption (paragraph 2–5). The inclusion about adoption is new and is an indication that NRT and adoption are perceived to be of the same order. (2) The preamble to the law states that the aim of the law is to secure that medical use of biotechnology is used in the best interest of human beings in a society where there is room for all (paragraph 1–1). The concern of the legislators with regard to assisted conception and the application of biotechnology in medicine is tied to the potentialities that these technologies represent regarding choice and possible eugenic practices. They want to avoid selection in the creation of desirable children. Phrased in positive terms, the law underscores an explicit value of equality, implicitly refuting the dangers of what has been termed a 'sorting society' (*sorteringssamfunnet*; see Solberg 2003; Melhuus 2005b). A 'sorting society' is understood to be a society that allows, even potentially, for any form of sorting of its members, and applied to NRT it refers directly to what may be termed a hierarchy of desirability with regard to the potential characteristics of the future child. All human life is in principle of equal value. This implies that permitting prenatal screening during the period when self determined abortion is still possible (the first twelve weeks of pregnancy) is considered unethical in so far as this opens the way for an abortion on the grounds of fetal defects. Thus, the law echoes the terms set by the 1956 Adoption Law, where only strong adoption was admitted: there is no turning back and couples must 'take what they get'. Today, prospective parents – adoptive or other – may not specify the desired qualities of their future child, such as sex, colour, abilities, etc.

Many of these issues were (and are) controversial, such as the continued prohibition on egg donation, the restrictions on prenatal screening and, to some extent, the revoking of donor anonymity. Different interested parties were variously engaged with these questions and, although it is interesting to pursue the different positions, in the context of this chapter we wish to draw attention to the most salient arguments relating to social and biological forms of belonging, the collapsing of rights and biogenetic origins with a notion of identity and the idea that Norwegian society is one 'where there is room for all'. However, before doing so, we shall return to adoption and the revision of the Adoption Law in 1986.

Adoption Laws 1986–99

The first major reconsideration of the 1917 Adoption Act resulted in a new act of 1986. As was the case in 1917 and 1956, this Adoption Law also came in the wake of a Children's Act (in this case that of 1981). The reason for a new law was the decline in infants available for domestic adoption and the near explosive growth of transnational adoption that was taking place in Norway during the 1970s and 1980s. The authorities saw it as urgent to bring transnational adoption under ordered and regulated control. Curiously, despite the concern about transnational adoption, the practice receives little explicit attention in the final act.

The 1986 Adoption Act is significant from many different perspectives. A reading between the lines reveals (yet again) a tension between biological and sociological thinking. Both biology and sociality (nature and nurture) receive attention in different sections of the text to the exclusion of each other. For example, legally speaking, adopted children are from now on to be regarded as in every way equal to biological children. This is in marked contrast to the attitudes held at the beginning of the twentieth century (as expressed in the 1917 law) and clearly reflects the growing concern for children's interests and child rights (Howell 2006). Moreover, the assumption is that adoptive parents will love and treat their adopted children as if they were their biological children, an assumption that runs contrary to what Demény (this volume) describes through her example of SOS foster mothers in Hungary. In Norway, there is no privileging of biological children.

A significant stipulation in the law is that adopted children should be told (if they so wish) the identity of their original parents upon reaching the age of legal maturity.[14] Thus, the post-war practice of anonymity – and hence secrecy – regarding biological origins of adoptees, which had led to a virtual taboo on the topic, was intentionally subverted. This provision, however, makes explicit an inherent ambiguity in the law: adoptees both are and are not equivalent to biological children. Moreover, it indicates a new emphasis being attributed to the relationship between biological relatives. At the same time, a change in the terminology used indicates a change in thinking from an exclusive biological set of values to a more sociological one. The words 'own children' (*egne barn*) and 'real parents' (*virkelige foreldre*) used in earlier laws were substituted with 'own borne children' (*egenfødte barn*) and 'original parents' (*opprinnelige foreldre*). This again stressed the fact that no differentiation was to be made between birth and adopted children.

The Adoption Law of 1986 and the first law regulating assisted conception in 1987 coincide in time. Yet it was not until 2003 that the provision in the Adoption Law granting the adopted child the right to know its biological origin was also incorporated into the law regulating assisted conception (explicitly by revoking donor anonymity, and implicitly by upholding the prohibition of egg donation). One of the arguments for abolishing the anonymity of sperm donors was precisely that of making the rights of donor children the same as the rights of adopted children. The fact that these are two very different ways of coming into being was unproblematically ignored, stressing rather that there should be no distinction between these two categories of children.

Two points are relevant here: first, the equating of adopted children with donor children (just as adopted children were equated with 'own children'); and secondly, the question of child rights has become central and is articulated through (if not reduced to) notions of identity understood as knowledge of biogenetic origin. Once again, aspects of adoption regulations are used to ground arguments relevant for assisted conception. Yet the emphasis is now on the child and its rights (to know his or her biogenetic origins, and hence his or her identity), irrespective of the parents, whether biogenetic, social or 'original'. Thus, we find that the concerns about origins iterated in the 1950s (that legislating anonymous sperm donation would create a general doubt about origins) are finally put to rest with the law of 2003. The biological foundations of kinship are formally acknowledged, both in the Adoption Law and in the law regulating assisted conception.

Conclusion

In this chapter, we have argued that adoption and assisted conception form a single universe of unnatural procreation and should therefore be treated as one discursive practice. We have suggested that these forms of 'unnatural' procreation are in the process of becoming naturalised and have indicated how this shift has come about. We have also shown that recent laws give precedence to biological bonds and that this reflects an increasing public preoccupation with biogenetics in the constitution of identity. In light of this, we return to the revelation about King Olav's conception and the fact that it did not give rise to moral outrage. Does this mean that laws do not reflect the opinions of the Norwegian public and that the power of kinning is more accepted by the Norwegian public than previously assumed to be the case? There is evidence that this is the case (Melhuus 2007).

We have discerned a number of similar preoccupations and solutions in legislation on adoption and NRT. However, the much older laws regulating adoption represent more than a mere background against which legislation concerning assisted conception can be understood. Rather, the evolving positions with regard to adoption represent indigenous cultural models through which assisted conception is interpreted and evaluated. Here, adoption becomes (paradoxically) a natural model against which other forms of unnatural procreation are measured. Not only is adoption a familiar phenomenon, it is also one that has been legally part of the public domain for almost a century. With artificial insemination by donor in the 1950s and in vitro fertilization in the early 1980s, established understandings of kinship were mobilised in order to make (moral) sense of these new procreative practices and the relationships they entailed. Alongside perceptions of natural procreation, adoption became a model employed in order to accommodate these totally new phenomena.

Adoption challenges biogenetic relatedness as a basis for creating kinship, while at the same time – unlike conception through donor gametes – adopted children are born in the familiar, natural manner. Adoption does not challenge the natural order. Adoption laws are based on a recognition of the difference between biological and social connectedness (see Cadoret, this volume, for an elaboration of the significance of this distinction). In fact, adoption articulates this fundamental difference and the inherent tension between them. Yet the cumulative result of the legislative process concerning adoption is that adopted children and birth children are the same in the eyes of the law. This also applies to those conceived by donor sperm. This idea of sameness is (and perhaps can only be) established through an accepted notion of the individual and his or her rights, coupled to the notion of the inherent equality of all humans regardless of origin.

The new reproductive technologies create confusion about what makes a relative in different ways from that of adoption. The fragmentation of procreation that takes place gives new meanings to eggs, sperm, wombs, gestation, birth, maternity and paternity. It is the need to establish some form of certainty that becomes critical, and the law is an attempt to cater to this need. The laws define the various kin relatives that become operative following an adoption or donor insemination.[15] In both cases, the law votes in favour of the intended parents in so far as they are defined as legal parents. At the same time, ambivalences with regard to biological origin prevail in so far as adopted children and donor children are given the right to find out about their biological parents upon reaching legal maturity if they so wish. Collapsing notions of biology and rights, knowledge of biological origin is considered to be in the best interest of the child, irrespective of the effect upon the other relationships that such knowledge might involve.

If adoption oscillates between 'original' and adopted parents, between biological and social parenthood, the distinctions are at least clear-cut and adopted family and kin relations are formed on an 'as if' basis. There is no doubt about the status or the origin of the child, even if the biological parents are not known. Assisted conception, however, interferes directly with what is perceived as the natural (f)act of procreation and herein lies the problem, at least for some Norwegian lawmakers.

Although we have argued that as acts of procreation, adoption and the use of donor sperm are perceived as analogically the same, the subsequent lives that adopted children and donor children live are very different. Transnational adoption is always public knowledge due to the fact that the children look different from their kin. This means that adoptive parents and their children have to cope with the fact that the nature of their relationship can never be hidden. This, however, is not the case for donor parents and their children.

Notes

This chapter is based on research carried on within three consecutive and overlapping research projects/programmes: 'Meanings of kinship in Norway' and 'The transnational flow of concepts and substances', financed by the Norwegian Research Council (NFR) and 'The Public Understanding of Genetics' (PUG), financed by the European Commission. We want to thank members of the PUG team for discussions and comments on our work throughout the period of the research programme. We especially want to thank the editors of this book for thoughtful comments on the first drafts of this chapter.

1. Dagbladet, http://www.dagbladet.no/?/nyheter/2004/10/14/411285.html.
2. *Timesonline*, 15 October 2004; article by Laura Peek.
3. There is a striking similarity between Laking's son, Guy Laking, and the late King Olav.
4. This is according to both a brief survey carried out by *Aftenposten* (Friday, 15 October 2004) and according to interviews with various well-known people as well as interviews with lay people (e.g. in *Dagsnytt 18*, a debate programme run by the Norwegian Broadcasting Corporation (NRK) five days a week).
5. However, this discourse has not yet been able to accommodate homosexuals and their perceived rights to have children, by either adoption or assisted conception. See Cadoret (this volume) for a further discussion on homosexual parenting in France.
6. For an interesting contrast to Spain, see Orobitg and Salazar (2005).
7. See Children's Act (Lov om barn og foreldre (barneloven) 1981–04, no. 7, chapter 2 (Who is the father of the child), § 6 (amended 20 December 2002, active from 1 April 2003, according to res. 20 des 2002 no. 1696).
8. Again there is an interesting contrast to Spain, where only the child, if he or she is over eighteen, or the mother acting on behalf of the child, can make such a request. The primacy of the best interests of the child is what presumably justifies this in Spain (Carles Salazar, personal communication). Moreover, the Norwegian case seems to substantiate Porqueres i Gené and Wilgaux's (this volume) suggestion that today's trend is to redefine the father as *quem sanguis demonstrant*, and can be interpreted as an attempt to make absent fathers present, or 'known', if only through establishing biogenetic connectedness (see Demény, this volume, for a discussion of the problems of the 'missing' father in Hungary).
9. The Abortion Law was passed in 1975 (Act of 13 June 1975, no. 50 om svangerskapsavbrudd) and amended in 1978 to allow for the right to self determination within the first twelve weeks (act of 16 June 1978, no. 66).
10. Adopsjonsloven av 1917: 'At knytte band'.
11. This was in line with the *pater est* rule, whereby a child born to a married woman automatically becomes the legal child of her husband. With the amendment in 1979 of the Law of Personal Names of 1964, a child had to be registered with a first name and a surname within six months of birth. The mother's or father's surname was equally acceptable. If no registration was made, the child would be given its mother's surname.
12. The reasons that it took so long to pass legislation are not easy to tease out. Partially they have to do with a failed Nordic initiative to coordinate policies regarding AID; partially they have to do with political processes in Norway and the fact that AID was a controversial issue and hotly contested (see Melhuus 2001, 2005a).

13. Act 2003–12–05–100. Lov om humanmedisinsk bruk av bioteknologi (bioteknologiloven).
14. The point about the right to know one's biological origins was a contentious issue in the formulation of the Hague Convention on Inter-country Adoption (1993). Whereas almost all receiving countries were in favour, most donor countries disagreed. Such a clause was not included.
15. This is also the case for those using IVF, as the law prohibits egg donation, insisting that the fertilised egg be returned to the womb from which it was taken; in this way 'mother' remains an unambiguous category.

CHAPTER 10

FIELDS OF POST-HUMAN KINSHIP

Ben Campbell

There is a strong current to the contributions in this volume, and much of the kinship and genetics literature, that the issue at hand is how contemporary families are being made and talked about in the light of DNA transmission, assisted reproductive technologies and their relationship to other 'non-natural' means of making family members, such as adoption. This chapter questions the assumptions that kinship broadly equates with the domain of human family connections, and that 'kinship and genetics' concern creative resolutions of genetic knowledge and familial contexts.

There is a strong assumption here about what kinship consists of anthropologically, as a subset of human relations tied to the domestic domain. Focusing on interpersonal family relatedness and kinship 'ways of thinking' privileges genealogical modes of reckoning and evaluating relationships. Even when importance is given to active practices that incorporate creative makings of family and relatedness (such as naming, feeding, and rituals of belonging), these are still embedded in a framework of how individuals are conceptually accommodated in networks and registers of human familiality and identity, which happen not to rely on direct genetic filiation. My argument is that kinship as a comparative enquiry needs to bring relations with non-humans into view, to explore 'kinship' dimensions beyond family connection. Genetic knowledge and technology reconfigure not only familial landscapes of information and reproductive choice, but also the relations between 'the human' and 'the natural'. Biologists use kinship to discuss the relationship of the human genome with that of other species, and to keep this apart from social anthropologists' use of it for differentiating conscious fields of social connection would be to accept rather than problematise the cosmology of naturalism (Descola 2005), where biologists' use of kinship refers to a knowable world of physical connection common to all life forms, separate from anthropological worlds of particular cultural meanings.

Comparative kinship studies have revealed numerous ways of connecting human and non-human worlds. Whether it is cattle with the Nuer (Evans-Pritchard 1940), pigs in Melanesia (Rappaport 1968, Strathern 1988) or consanguine plants and affinal prey in Amazonia (Descola 1996), human kinship has been enfolded in wider relations with the non-human world. Urbanised Euro-American society is clearly more detached from regular non-human convivialities (pet-keeping is popular but optional), but to neglect non-human interactions in ideas of kinship would be to miss out on perspectives for thinking anthropologically about kinship and genetics. At the origins of modern kinship theory, Feeley-Harnik comments that L.H. Morgan 'used "breed", "cross", "half-breed", and "quarter-breed" as if he were talking about his family's herd of wool bearers' (2001: 58). In the Great Lakes area, people would speak of their kinship and marriage, and be telling Morgan simultaneously of beaver kinship, in ways that 'intimately entwined fates of human and other creatures' (ibid: 80). Genomic comparisons now bring the human and non-human back into relation. The uniqueness or exceptionalism of human ontology and Euro-American kinship is given new problematics by genetics, and provides grounds for thinking comparatively about how kinship cosmologically locates the human in the world. It is not just in new ways of making and thinking about families that genetics transforms understandings of kinship, but in reflection on new kinds of intentional agency in a world where the boundaries of species and their interrelations have become subject to unprecedented kinds of human intervention.

By including non-humans in kinship perspectives, connections are made with discussions of 'post-human' society. I use the British media's response in 2003 to the scientific findings of the nationwide investigation into likely environmental consequences of growing genetically modified crops in the UK to claim that a relation of protective kinship between people and the non-human inhabitants of the landscape was discovered in this moment. A latent connectivity between people and the environment was revealed on the verge of its irreversible conversion into a resource for biotechnological farming. If we had thought that modern European kinship had shed any kind of extra-human cultural dependency, like the Nuer's vis-à-vis cattle, and only entertained metaphorical conceits in anthropomorphic narratives (from Beatrix Potter to Bug's Life), the prospect of genetically modified cropping systems and the possibility of feral recombinant DNA stalking the hedgerows provoked a response of solidarity in the British media with the creatures of the countryside.

I use the term 'post-human' to mark changes in how the human can now be talked about with knowledge of the human genome and the use of genetics to restructure interactions with other species. The category of human and its relation to the non-human are changed by the prospect of germ-line engineering and DNA transfer across lines of species and phyla. Technologically mediated reproduction evokes explicit reflexivity on the autonomy of a natural world. Reproduction has been brought out of a naturalised black box of assumed processes and contexts of control. A circumspect anthropology for the new politics of human and non-human fertility moves kinship beyond strictly internal 'human' concerns of relatedness. Novel opportunities for assisted choice in having children and in designing the genetic agency of food crops create a contested stage for the regulatory powers that strategically close down certain kinds of option. No longer are humans passive in the face of the genetic lottery of hereditary accident, nor are they situated at a distance from a self-reproducing realm of nature beyond human activity (Strathern 1992a). It is the new configuration of possible life relations, and the move beyond the Enlightenment clarity of exceptional, human conscious agency over an inert nature, that warrants the 'post' in question.

What Kinship is All About

Recent attempts to recover anthropology's claims to kinship expertise have included Franklin and McKinnon's (2001) interrogation of the ways that new kinds of family relatedness are growing in contemporary processes of social change around the world and in the face of new technological possibilities. Their overview extends from 'kinning' as a process of domesticating difference in the cultural heritage of adoptees in international adoption (Howell 2001), to the use of kinship as a term for characterising connections with analogical resemblances to human relatedness, such as in human – machine hybrids (Helmreich 2001).

In their valuable treatment, Franklin and McKinnon have not entirely escaped an implicit curiosity for 'what kinship is all about' (Schneider 1984). Although they take us through a host of 'contingent and productive' (Franklin and McKinnon 2001: 7) contexts and conceptual linkages, there remains a sense that kinship with its 'substantial codings' is about an area of social enclosure, congealed through embodiment, to do with 'shared kind' and familial closeness. This was in previous generations substantialised by anthropologists as 'the domestic domain' (Goody 1976), and embraced the household, the family and the private as a coherent relational field in opposition to the public domain, where contrasting principles of sociality and exchange could be recognised.

With structuralist exchange theory, an alternative view of the domestic was offered that started not from the primacy of descent, but from extra-domestic reciprocities in the reproduction of the domestic through ongoing affinity. The presence of the reproductive exchange relation and the affinal other within the minimal unit of kinship configure the domestic as already in articulation with alliances between types of difference. In the structuralist formulation, non-humans figure only as elements that are good for thinking with, neglecting exchanges of less cerebral flows that bring non-humans into sociality: for instance, with life forms that respond through evolutionary domestication to our embodied relations with the world.[1] Jones argues that, after hunters turned to arrows rather than spears:

> Wolves – dogs as they became – became more useful as they would chase and pull down wounded prey. Such a creature took at once a large step toward the fireside ... At Ein Mallah in Israel, in a grave of the earliest farmers, is the skeleton of a puppy buried next to a child. A wild animal had become a member of the family. Soon its muzzle shrank, its teeth became smaller, its eye grew large and round, and the modern dog had arrived. (Jones 2000: 34)

In contrast to 'kin', the terms 'family' and 'household' more readily include animal associations, as productive domestic assets, or as pets that can be seen as complementary members in families of affection, even as subjects substituting for human relatives. Against modern understandings that would restrict 'kin' only to other humans, Haraway (1997) uses kinship provocatively to place us as relational beings in an encounter with the strange productions of biotechnological capitalism. She invites us to think about the kinship we might have with them, in terms of concern for the relatedness of life, especially if we take account of their hybrid bioinformatic lineages and their confounding of conventional categories of being and object.

Such apparent projections of the language of kinship to the non-human or to human-animated entities are no longer so easily contained within the dualism of literal or metaphorical connection. Genetic knowledge, whether of human relations or modified organisms opens up areas of instability between the literal and the metaphorical. Anthropologists working in this field have charted the processes of normalisation or purification that people have shown in giving strategically conventional shape to biological facts (Thompson 2001), or have explored the pressure exercised by hybrid entities on notions of life and kinship (Helmreich 2001).

Descola (2005) offers an ambitious, comparative typology for relations between the human and non-human. In his category of modern naturalism, a cosmology that presents the world out there as a mute, physical unity is set against the species-unique quality of human conscious agency. For Descola, artificial intelligence or the recognition of human-like intelligence among higher primates only emphasises the human-centric properties of this scheme. His point is to emphasise the distinctiveness of this cosmology in comparative terms and to warn against its inappropriate extension to understand the relations of humans and non-humans in other societies that 'have not hesitated to invite into the concert of their social life the most modest of plants, and the most insignificant of animals' (my translation, Descola 2005: 15). A problem with his approach is that he compares Amazonian hunters and cultivators with the great thinkers of the Enlightenment, to the exclusion of other modern coevals, who appear in the work of Feeley-Harnik (2001, n.d.) to have furnished the foundational modern thinkers for the study of kinship (Morgan) and evolution (Darwin) with some of their most potent images, in apparent defiance of human exceptionalism. Taking kinship beyond the human and beyond the literalism of genetic substance as defining relatedness, arguments can be made for thinking outside the cosmology of naturalism and in terms of relational universes of intimate responsibility that cross the human/non-human divide. The prospect of displacing ecological communities and their iconic songbirds with genetically modified crops challenged vernacular, analogical relatedness across species.

Genetically Modified Crops and the Kinship of Life

To track biotechnology's relational pathways, I use kinship in a very broad sense, as a technology for the organisation of solidarities, desire and exchange, not confined to specifically human domains of reference, to analyse the British media's reception of the scientific evaluation of genetically modified organisms.

In the mounting controversy over GMOs in Europe from the mid-1990s, people gave many reasons for opposing these crops' introduction into the food chain.[2] These ranged from 'tampering with nature' and lack of labelling information about product content for consumers to concern about multinational control over the world food supply. In terms of World Trade Organisation agreements, the only legal basis for resisting GMOs was evidence of harm to human health or the environment. The British government's scientific advice suggested minimal health implications. To complement a public opinion consultation exercise held in 2003, a decision was made to examine the crops scientifically for environmental impact. 'Farm-scale evaluations' (FSE) on over 200 farms across the country looked for three years at the effects of growing crops modified for herbicide resistance on plants, insects and birds in field locations. The results were published on 16 October 2003 and were widely reported and discussed by the press.

Media reporting is obviously designed to impact on cultural nerve endings. A notable reverence for the details of the findings as scientifically objective is apparent, but latent, analogically social readings are simultaneously emergent. Even in the decontextualisation of the facts from public concerns about GMOs, these latent readings invoke missing relationships of people to agricultural environments. The newspapers play on an iconic cultural status of birds, with their lyrical-sounding vernacular names, and the interdependence of life forms under threat from dosings of weedkiller which, only by implication, include humans. In the public debate, where socio-political arguments over the technology were hierarchically displaced by legal and scientific authority, the birds, weeds and mini-beasts can be seen to stand analogically for human presence. All the weight of social concerns about GMOs now hung in the environmental basket.

On 17 October 2003, the *Independent* (a centre-left newspaper) front-page headline declared, 'Proven: the Environmental Dangers that may Halt GM Revolution'. The Farm-scale evaluations confirmed 'conservationists' concerns that the GM crops scheduled for growth in Britain would mean yet another blow for the insects, flowers and birds that have been decimated by more than 30 years of intensive farming'. In its inside-page report, Chris Pollock, chairman of the FSE scientific steering committee, drew attention to the uniqueness of this research, which sought to anticipate the effects of cultivating the new crops: 'It is the first time a novel agricultural technology has been trialled extensively before it has been introduced rather than us examine the consequences after it has been introduced' (*Independent* 17 October 2003: 4).

I shall concentrate on three themes of the media reporting of the results. One is the picture of biodiversity in field ecology that emerged from the trials, the second is the consideration given to the desirability for people and society of further intensification of farming, and the third is an issue the trials did not address, but which most of the newspapers could not leave alone – the prospect of cross-pollination from GM crops with 'wild relatives'.

Many newspapers presented factual findings adjacent to commentary. The *Daily Telegraph* (right-wing) provided a 'question and answer' section, where 'What did they discover? was answered: 'GM oilseed rape and GM beet damaged the environment. There were fewer butterflies, bees and invertebrates because there were 80% fewer weeds and seeds for them to eat' (*Daily Telegraph*, 17 October 2003: 3). The *Guardian* (centre-left) had a section 'Birds and bees: how wildlife suffered', itemising the different outcomes for a range of species under GM and conventional farming. A previously little researched creature the springtail, a small wingless arthropod, was one of the few species that seemed to benefit under GM oilseed rape, due to the timing of weedkiller application and the amount of decaying plant matter available to it.

The Times ('establishment') countryside editor described the results as painting 'a grim picture of a landscape denuded of many farmland birds, butterflies, insects, and common field plants', and a Royal Society for the Protection of Birds spokesman was quoted as saying that GM crops could mean 'the final nail in the coffin for some species' (*The Times*, 17 October 2003: 9). The tabloid, right-wing *Daily Mail* declared: 'farming the so-called Frankenstein crops risks creating a biological desert by wiping out wild plants, butterflies, bees and birds' (*Daily Mail*, 17 October 2003: 6–7). The *Guardian* pronounced that the further deprivation of habitat and food from birds and animals would be 'an irreplaceable loss to the countryside which once teemed with the sights and sounds of creatures on and above the ground' (The *Guardian* 17 October 2003: 1). The editorial in the *Independent* noted the finding that 'Fewer weeds means fewer – and fewer varieties of – insects, and that in turn means fewer corn buntings, skylarks and yellowhammers' (*Independent* 17 October 2003: 20). The *Guardian* reported that governmental responses 'were cautious', but the Environment Minister Elliott Morley was quoted as saying 'GM crops had severe implications for birds.' In the chorus of doom it was left to Paul Rylott from the industry body promoting GM to argue 'scaremongering is not supported by the facts' and claims that the crops would 'wipe out wildlife' were unfounded (*Independent* 17 October 2003: 5).

What has all this to do with kinship? Let us take 'severe implications for birds'. The creatures themselves are not going to consciously deliberate the consequences of GM oilseed rape, beet and maize, but 'implication' and its cognates 'imply' and 'implicate' in my dictionary bring up 'entwine together', 'enfold', 'involve', 'entangle', 'express indirectly' and 'insinuate'. The implications are for people to consider on behalf of the birds, in the knowledge about the likely avian outcomes of intensified applications of weedkiller in the fields. Herbicide-tolerant GMO cultivation would more efficiently convert sunlight into plant growth, to the greater advantage of human food crops against weed competition and the wildlife that depends on the weeds. It is the human senses that register 'irreplaceable loss', 'grim picture' and the series of deprivations along the food chain from weeds through insects to birds, whose names carry cultural genealogies evocative of pastoral symphonies and Shakespearean sonnets. It is to human ears and eyes that disappearing sights and sounds will matter. Radcliffe-Brown's totemic question 'Why all these birds?' might be asked here, and, as Lévi-Strauss put it, 'The connexion is not arbitrary, nor is it a relation of contiguity' (1973: 147). What kinds of extra-species solidarities, desires and exchanges are called forth in the brute demonstration of impending biodiversity decline? I shall take this up later.

Faced with a decisive moment in the extent to which British field ecology should be dedicated to the cause of maximised efficiency in farming practices, priorities of culturally determined value enter the frame. The left-leaning Mirror tabloid newspaper used dramatic headlines to emphasise the choice, borrowing the title of Rachel Carson's book as its main statement 'Silent Spring', continuing with 'Birds and Bees: Technology v Wildlife'. The *Independent*'s editorial writer was clear about the alternatives now presented to decision makers:

> the choice comes down to enhanced yields versus reduced biodiversity. Broadly, that is the choice that has been offered by intensive farming since the Industrial Revolution. And there has been a growing recognition in recent decades that farming policy should be tending in the opposite direction to that offered by today's genetically modified crops. The movement should be away from intensive farming and towards the preservation of biodiversity. You do not have to be a 100 per cent organic enthusiast to appreciate that the environmental costs of modern farming methods are too high. (*Independent*, 17 October 2003: 20)

The *Guardian*'s account of the trial results sets the government's policies for promoting biotechnology against other pledges made to protect the environment. Chief among these was the aim of reversing the loss of bird life in the countryside, which the government had identified as a 'quality of life' indicator (meaning human life). It quoted David Gibbons (a panel member of the farm-scale evaluations) saying the results were 'dramatic' in the evidence that '[t]here will be less food for birds' (*Guardian*, 17 October 2003: 4).

The science journalist Andy Coghlan, writing in the *New Scientist*, observed that in contrast to the balance of farming and wildlife in UK and Europe, farmers in the US and Australia use powerful broad-spectrum weedkillers to create 'fields sterilised of everything except the crop. Farmland there is purely for business, and if people want to see wildlife, they can visit national parks. But in Europe, farmland is used for leisure as well as producing food, and conservationists want farmers to be kinder to what wildlife remains' (*New Scientist*, 18 October 2003: 8). Coghlan added that the UK has witnessed a 'catastrophic decline' in a number of bird species since the Second World War, with modern agriculture's expansion of field sizes at the expense of hedgerows, the use of agrochemicals and the increase in winter crops, which remove fallow sequences.

Counter arguments were presented in the conservative *Daily Telegraph*. Its editorial contended that risks from GM crops were no greater than with what had happened with 'conventional crops over the last 9,000 years', and that anti-GM 'feeling' is simply motivated by 'fear of the new' (*Daily Telegraph*, 17 October 2003: 27). The *Independent*'s show of balanced coverage included the claim from Paul Rylott of the Agriculture Biotechnology Council that 'this evidence reiterates commercial experience from around the world, that GM crops are more flexible and can enhance biodiversity' (*Independent*, 17 October 2003: 5). Key to this argument was the finding that, of the crops trialled, growing GM maize was less damaging to wildlife than 'conventional' maize, which required especially powerful weedkillers.

The *Daily Mail* quoted the Environment Minister Elliot Morley restating the legally determined position regarding withdrawal of approval for the new crops: 'GM crops can only be grown if they get consent. Whether they get consent depends on whether there are environmental impacts' (*Daily Mail*, 17 October 2003: 6). Anthropologists will be interested to see how the social aspects of technology assessment become compartmentalised as separate from environmental ones. The effects of this boundary making are powerful in giving priority to scientific realism, which establishes as more solidly reliable a foundational domain of nature and biology, which can also be recognised as operating in the area of assisted human reproduction. As with the latter, one might expect to find all manner of relational enfoldings, entwinings and entanglements of tactics and representations that blur dichotomous views of nature and culture. In this area, Edwards (this volume) draws attention to 'boundary objects', whose ambivalent relationship to purified versions of nature or culture provides people with opportunities for innovative practices of living and 'kinning'. Another effect of the enforced compartmentalisation of environmental truth and value fenced off from relationships of social and political 'domains' is to let loose symbolic inflections of the environmental as implying narratives of the social and political in analogical refractions of moral responsibility. Issues of metaphor and likenesses of kinship will be taken up later.

The final component to think about in the media stories is transgenic pollination. Here we see the pollen spores of modified crops seeking out relatives in the British countryside. The farm-scale evaluations had not actually investigated this dimension of GM crops, but a study from the Department of Environment and Rural Affairs had just been published before the FSE report. It had found that GM pollen from oilseed rape had travelled distances of over 25 km, and would be likely to cross-fertilize with *Brassica rapa*, the wild turnip or 'bargeman's cabbage' (*Farmer's Guardian*, 17 October 2003: 7). It is these modified genes going 'feral' and roaming freely to breed with native species that have prompted talk in the newspapers of herbicide- or insect-resistant 'superweeds'. The *Farmer's Guardian* quoted a Friends of the Earth spokesperson: 'We would be starting a huge outdoor experiment' (ibid.: 7). In contrast to 'alarmist' interpretations, an industry spokesman said the research on cross-pollination 'merely confirms well-documented evidence that natural hybridisation between the species occurs at very low levels' (ibid.: 7).

In recognising that some GM crops have evolutionary relatives and that genetically compatible alliances could be made 'in nature' beyond the intentions of biotechnological design (with the modified genes giving rise to consequences in species' evolution bearing the trace of human selected traits), the language of kinship used by geneticists and anthropologists is commingled. Biotechnologists, as evidenced by the spokesman quoted above, oscillate between the familiar normalising language of biology as the routine inevitability of life processes and the transformational artifice of using genetic traits in novel combinations to human advantage. Haraway remarks that transgenic organisms 'simultaneously fit into well established taxonomic and evolutionary discourses and also blast widely understood senses of natural limit' (1997: 56). Further, she pursues the substantialised power and hybrid agency of recombinant DNA life forms, commenting that 'refiguration of the kinship between different orders of life, the generative splicing of synthetic DNA and money produces promising genetic fruit' (Haraway 1997: 66). Her use of 'kinship' both mocks continuing ideological assumptions of naturalness and draws attention to how the reproduction of humans, creatures and machine life has shifted beyond conventional parameters of fertility.

In biotechnology's discourse of GM crops not endangering biodiversity at large, insisting on the 'substantial equivalence' of GM and conventional foods and arguing against the need for boundaries to limit cross-contamination with non-GM or organic farms, it argued for a case-by-case assessment of the new crops, rather than a verdict on GM per se. To deny the possibility of GM plants' sexual reproduction with wild relatives is comparable to strategies of kinship 'truncation', noticed in practices of selective solidarity. The motive of denying kinship with wild plants, of arguing that the transgenic crops are containable for human purposes and will not form hybrid kin associations, is a recognisable 'officializing strategy' (Bourdieu 1977) to privilege certain networks of relatedness over others.

The media's treatment of the release of the farm-scale evaluations was noticeably deferential to the language of science. (It was mostly left to the cartoonists to bring out more imaginative and transgressive views of how nature, society, money and politics were simultaneously at play in the process of assessing GM crops.) Such was the effectiveness of separating out environmental science from 'ethical' and 'economic' categories of public concern that statements about 'less food for birds' were not contextualised within the register of science, by arguments that the hungry of the world needed feeding. (These arguments resurfaced when government decisions were taken.) The newspapers dramatised the science of wildlife loss, but did not explore the relationship of field ecology and society, other than as a choice about economic or biodiversity values. Ecological science was imagined to speak for itself or to stand as a view on what was happening 'out there', with the issue of people's relationship to the landscape silently contained. This could reflect the distance of protected authenticity by which Descola (1996, 2005) has characterised Western relationships of 'naturalism' towards the environment. Science was very effectively kept apart from any visibility of emotional or other relational connections people might have with springtails, skylarks or corn buntings. The environment was there to be seen and taken in as a contained and knowable system, but it missed the element of human presence, apart from tractor drivers, or commentators with a scientific or economic stake.

It thus appeared as the introduction of a different order of knowledge when a personalised human dimension of interactive and subjective presence relating to this threatened ecology cropped up in a corner of the media. It came in the figure of Les Firbank, the scientific leader of the farm-scale evaluations. Interviewed in the *New Scientist*, he revealed a kinship connection with the British farming landscape. Raised on a small farm in the county of West Yorkshire, his PhD was a study of the population dynamics of an arable weed (the corncockle). He described his family's direct experience of ecological change:

> I can remember a period when I was a kid in Yorkshire when we had cowslips all over the farm. By the time I was 10 most of them had gone. We thought it was just one of those things. We had no idea it was because of the way we were managing the land. We had put too much manure on it. As a family we didn't want to do any harm. That issue – how to balance farming and wildlife – has always driven my research interests. (*New Scientist*, 25 October 2003: 46)

So at last a human dimension that involves a very conventional 'kinship' – a family with a livelihood of interaction with fields, animals and plants – is made to appear as key to the motivation of the chief scientist, which enfolds, entwines and entangles a scientist's reflexive practice with a relational context of human and non-human conviviality. The *Scotsman* newspaper encapsulated a conscientious relationship to the farming landscape by using an old-fashioned English term of ethically instrumental kinship with the land – 'good husbandry'.

Discussion

As Firbank and others made clear, it was really the herbicides that were on trial for their environmental harm, rather than the crops modified to resist them. The genes were only part of a weedkiller management package, whose impact on a range of environmental issues, such as protection of birds and organic farming, constructed particular lines of opposition. Issues of boundaries and their transgression (between nature and society, GM and non-GM, profit and biodiversity) loomed large in these debates, and confirm Franklin's insistence on looking at 'boundary work' performed in the maintenance of kinship, gender and 'the marketing of these lines, species, and families of products' (2001: 315). The biotechnology industry and the organic certification business are equally involved in the politics of redefining commodities, consumer wishes, markets and nature. Boundaries are not present without categorical labour to make them evident, and boundaries of different orders play off each other: from criteria of food labelling to crop planting limits drawn on the ground. It was noticeable how the image of Britain as a 'small, windy island', with a closely interdependent farmland and human population, served to differentiate topologies for intensive agriculture between the US with its vast, open prairies and UK conditions. The territorial mosaic of farmland and wildlife habitat use purposes in the UK was too mixed up for any simple implementation of protective separation distances between GM and non-GM.

My argument is that an extra-human relatedness (a kin-like analogy) was actualised in the conflict over GMOs, when food production for humans was presented starkly as a lethal loss of food for biodiversity. When people were confronted with the prospect of a diminished 'nature' that was no longer autonomous and when the regenerative capacity of the soil and the creatures living from it was made negotiable and brought into a deliberative public sphere, latent solidarities of interest projected across the human/non-human divide. The 'kinship' resonances of GMOs have to be recovered from noises and silences. The media's response to knowledge about threats to farmland wildlife respected the narrative power of scientific expertise in descriptions of the natural food chain. The newspapers were entranced by this depiction of another world, which humans could appreciate at a relation of respectful distance. The lay-expert divide appeared to be credible in a moment of awe displayed in the face of the extent and content of what the research had discovered. But the scientific frame did not for long hold the discursive bounds of the debate over GM. Four months later, Clare Devereux of the Five-year Freeze coalition commented: 'The government just does not get it. The public is way ahead in understanding that agricultural biotechnology is about a lot more than just the science. It is about livelihoods, choice, culture, the biodiversity of our landscape, the survival of small farmers – and GM crops could potentially threaten all of these' (*Guardian*, 20 February 2004: 8).

Earlier, I touched on the debate about totemism in anthropology. Clearly, the relationship of wildlife to people in contemporary Britain is not operating on the same kind of grounds as is found in kinship practices organising moiety affinities around non-human identity hooks.[3] What kind of otherings and proximity with the non-human can instead be discussed?

Lévi-Strauss (1973) presented so-called totemic phenomena as a variety of ways for organising relations between people via languages of non-human differentiation (it was the differences between differences of kind that resembled each other). Metonymic identifications are not the issue – with totemism or GMO opposition. But nor will 'metaphorical' kinship serve the purpose of the argument here. For Ingold (1996), metaphor depends on a pre-structured separation of nature from culture that fails to attend to how people and environments interact. Human affinities with the natural world are more than tokens of signifying convention.

The birds, butterflies and bees of UK farmland, I would argue, became in a process of implication the imagined community of the British people. Their presence and their relationships of countryside interaction haunt the gaps in the reporting of the scientific evaluations, through a long-standing cultural and scientific relationship with field ecology. Pertinent here is the image of the 'entangled bank' that Darwin referred to in *The Origin of Species*, with its 'singing, flittering flow of creatures' and their 'hidden bonds of descent' (cited in Feeley-Harnik 2003: 318). Feeley-Harnik asks again Radcliffe-Brown's question when pondering the totemic puzzle, 'Why all these birds?' His answers, she argues, were overly socio-centric, neglecting the cross-species bonds of sociality. The importance of birds to Darwin (e.g. Galapagos finches, and the genealogy of the European rock dove) came from an interest in the intimate kinship between humans and birds in con-social dwelling. In particular it was the rearing of 'fancy' pigeon breeds by hand-loom silk weavers in London and their expert eyes for selecting the iridescence of plumage for trait enhancement that provided Darwin with the idea of modifying the weavers' 'artificial selection' to become his 'natural selection'.

Feeley-Harnik (2003) argues that since before Darwin's time there has been a sensitivity to biogeographical change through avian imagery, in which birds have acted as significant markers of transforming ecologies.

(Remember the Labour government had made birds a 'quality of life indicator'.) I imagine people in boardrooms of biotech companies after the trials asking Radcliffe-Brown's question, 'Why all these birds?' The farm ecology on which the GM evaluations were performed was a social terrain on which the British and their multinational corporate cousins would have to negotiate over their novel plant familiars' rights for co-residence ('in a small island'). The acceptability of laboratory-modified, vegetable quasi-cousins was here linked to the fate of soil organisms, wild seed dispersal and the survival within agri-culture of fat hen, springtails, corn buntings and skylarks.

Science can be a form of politics by other means (Latour 2004), but its power lies in presenting a world of fact beyond particular value perspectives. As social, cultural and other consequences of GM farming were credited less authority for policymaking than scientific evidence, the creatures of farmland biodiversity substituted to make a sociality of life, photosynthesis and controlled ecological competitiveness acquire a narrative of moral-political judgement about changing times. The subliminal substitution of British rural (human) communities and wider consumers for the fate under biotech management of the mini-beasts, bugs, and weeds is more than a metaphorical association. The GM crop trials reactivated an old relationship of mutual attendance between people and birds, but now in terms of the language of technological choice or the deliberative 'share' between agriculture and biodiversity.

There is no single British or even English cultural relationship with birds and the countryside, and indeed the important fact is the diversity of actors and discourses contending with each other in environmental politics. The anti-GM coalition ranged from Prince Charles, mainstream conservation organisations and neo-pagans through to anti-capitalists. However, as a general cultural process, a permeability of the language of care, protection and nurturance across the human/non-human divide is on the increase. This is apparent in the transfer of the language of compassionate 'adoption' to non-humans (gorillas, whales, etc.). An antivivisection campaign poster in 2006 features a laboratory monkey's face beneath a plea for 'Next of Kin'. To non-British people, this can appear to be a distinctive national attitude. The film-maker Kusturica made a kinship analogy, angered about a scene cut by the British censor, where a cat attacked a pigeon. A journalist put to him that 'You don't realize what an emotive issue pigeons are in England.' Kusturica responded:

> 'Was [the censor] brought up by pigeons or something?' He continued, 'What is the problem with you English? You killed millions of Indians and Africans, and yet you go nuts about the circumstances of the death of a single Serbian pigeon. I am touched you hold the lives of Serbian birds so dear, but you are crazy. I will never understand how your minds work.'
> (*Guardian*, 4 March 2005)

Conclusion

In talking about post-human kinship my purpose has been to recognise the junctures of human fertility history, and to talk of a parallel realisation that the way anthropologists have pursued the question of 'What is kinship all about?' in the West has tended to ignore the value of looking at how kinship is not simply about humans. Even if divides are maintained in a common-sense way between humans and non-humans, both the contexts in which human kinship is lived out and the consideration given to animals and plants as adjuncts, instruments and embodiments of familial intentionality deserve recognition. Kinship always needs to be placed in context, including those involving non-human interactions. Otherwise relatedness is ideologically divorced from the embodied conditions in which terms of connection are actually lived: the activities of making a home, caring for relatives through affection bestowed on kinspeople's pets, and the symbolic work performed by celebrating, for example, home-produced food, taking a 'family walk' in a country park or visiting a place where a relative grew up. If the comparative study of kinship is not to be confined to culturally specific definitions, it deserves to be viewed as a creative technology for making relations of solidarity, desire and exchange.

Whereas kinship served in modern anthropology to differentiate the internal organisation of disparate systems of sociocultural reproduction, the contexts in which relatedness now operates demand new parameters of thought. Arguments about the naturalised grounding of kinship in biology, as Franklin (2001) points out, need to take account of how biology has shifted. How biology offers resources for thinking who we are (both as social actors and as anthropologists) and how we understand our interactions as substantial flows with effects on hosts of humans and non-humans bring relational subjectivity in confluence with governance, technology, social movements and the global economy.

GM evaluation in the UK produced a refracted illumination of these relations, made visible through their opacity in a biological vision of the non-human world in suspension from directly human concerns. It was a suspension made possible by a combination of the authority of science to speak disinterestedly (and to surprise expectations), with the notion of the ecosystem as a measurable system of relations. GM technology was assessed for its impact on the non-human environment to make informed decisions about environmental implications for birds and people. Ecosystem biology managed a containment of technological cause and effect within a strictly material world, to produce a prediction of consequences to be subsequently processed through evaluative systems of a different order: global food politics, social demands for countryside protection and concerns for the survival of non-GM farming. Human exceptionalism to the natural world was thus instantiated in terms of what could be impartially known, distinct from processes of deciding on GM technology that were situated within a domain of competing and contingent values. In these respects it would hardly be possible to find as clear an example of Descola's (2005) cosmology of modern naturalism. It is the incompleteness of the naturalist ontology to account for the responses of extra-human connection evidenced by the newspapers' reporting of the GM trials, that makes the idea of a human exceptionalist cosmology hard to sustain.

My central point has been to suggest that this starkly dimorphic organisation of knowledge for technological governance produced conditions for analogical identifications across the human/non-human divide. The vision of imperilled wildlife was met with a reciprocal articulation of ethical responsibility. While there are possibilities for anthropological explanation of this response within what has conventionally been taken as kinship (for instance, the con-social intimacies of Darwin's weaver families and their doves, or the experience of land-family relationships revealed by the farm trials coordinator Les Firbank), I want to emphasise how genetic knowledge of humans, non-humans and human modified organisms re-situates how we can think of ourselves relationally to the non-human world.

The impact of genetic knowledge and technology has been frequently described in hyperbolic language. Woolfson, for instance, proclaims that, with the discovery of the evolutionary process through genetic variation, '[I]n an instant, the erosion of mankind's innocence was complete' (2004: 46). In his book *An Intelligent Person's Guide to Genetics*, he also concludes:

> If every aspect of our behaviour is shaped to some extent by our genetic programming, artificial modifications of these programs should enable key aspects of ourselves – including our shape, lifespan, intelligence, sense of equality, capacity for compassion, love, sexuality, empathy, aesthetics, justice and morality, all once assumed to be inviolable aspects of our humanity – to be modified or reconfigured from first principles. (Ibid.: 204)

My angle is to suggest that confident human exceptionalism, as species-specific biological, moral and subjective alterity to the rest of nature, is over, even if not in the mechanistic terms Woolfson proposes. This prompts us to look at our shared genomic similarities with other species, and our continuing influence on the evolution of non-human organisms (Pollan 2001), as well as the increasing possibilities for tweaking the normal flow of fertility events. Evidence for fractured boundaries of the human comes in the multiple arenas where boundary making of human and non-human is now being asserted. The UK's Human Fertilisation and Embryology Act, for example, has several references to experimental hamster fertilisation and embryology, and the legal requirement not to let more than a minimal number of cells develop. But, in artistic works too, the moral exceptionalism of humanity in relation to animals has become a theme that is being examined in radical ways, for instance, in terms of analogies between genocide and the treatment of animals (Coetzee 1999) and in terms of sexuality (Albie 2004).[4]

The 'End of History' author Fukuyama uses genetics to berate leftist thought for imagining infinite possibilities for people to change the conditions they are born into, but argues that history is, after all, continuing with genetic advances. His worry is that:

> biotechnology will cause us in some way to lose our humanity – that is, some essential quality that has always underpinned our sense of who we are and where we are going, despite all of the evident changes that have taken place in the human condition through the course of history. Worse yet, we might make this change without recognizing that we had lost something of great value. We might thus emerge on the other side of a great divide between human and posthuman history and not even see that the watershed had been breached because we lost sight of what that essence was. (Fukuyama 2002: 101)

Fukuyama (a proponent of regulation) and Woolfson (an inevitablist),[5] fill the analysis of the future with machines and protected essences. My argument is that neither machine nor essence encapsulates what being a human is all about, and that, rather than the question 'Who is a relative?', the question 'How do I relate to you?' (whether staring in the eyes of an IVF infant, at a goat, or at a genetically modified tomato on the supermarket shelf) will continue to perplex and produce differentiation in new and unpredictable ways. This framing points kinship in the direction of asking how and for what purposes people are making analogies and solidarities with other beings, and how genetic and relational discourses are articulated or muted in competing knowledge registers when a particular conflict becomes characterised as centred on genetics. For Descola, genetics has cosmologically enhanced the scientifically knowable unity of the external physical world, while human interiorities generate an unmanageable diversity of value systems. In this chapter I have attempted to demonstrate recalcitrant analogical connections among moderns. Despite Descola's naturalist cosmology: (1) they have practices of family and relational identity that confound the brute segregation of human and non-human; and (2) the prospect of reduced wildlife in genetically modified agriculture evinced a co-citizenship (contra Descola 2005. 542) with non-human others in a post-exceptional image. This was not so much the 'lost innocence' that Descola speaks of, but a new visualisation of relationships that drags the silent nature of naturalism from its condition of mute insentience (admittedly by excessive human interventions) and now asks what kind of ties with the population of 'the inanimate' might be envisaged.

Notes

1. 'We too cast unconscious evolutionary votes every time we reach for the most symmetrical flower or the longest French fry' (Pollan 2001: 262).

2. For an excellent treatment of the European contexts for opposition to GMOs, see Bauer and Gaskell (2002). Wynne (2001) gives an incisive analysis of the basis for public mistrust of UK institutions intended to communicate scientific advice. Lezaun (2004) analyses the different approaches to marketing GM products and consumer research in generating scepticism about multinationals' motives.
3. See Wagner (1977) for an analysis of one such kinship system in New Guinea, which takes 'analogical' flows of ideas about care and responsibility to explain the work of maintaining appropriate distinctions between categories of kin.
4. Edward Albie's (2004) play *The Goat or 'Who is Sylvia?'* explores aspects of innocence and horror in a man's revealed love for a goat, and the limits to the tolerance of desire within a modern family.
5. Woolfson comments, 'The largely irrational urge to preserve our current incarnation unchanged is no different from wanting to keep red telephone boxes or milkmen' (2004: 207).

CHAPTER 11

ARE GENES GOOD TO THINK WITH?

Carles Salazar

Tout ce que les linguistes nous avaient appris sur le langage, et qui semblait être sa propriété exclusive, nous nous apercevions que cela existe au cœur même de la matière vivante; que le code génétique et le code verbal présentent les mêmes caractéristiques et fonctionnent de la même façon. (Lévi-Strauss 1988: 149)

One of the aims of the research that has led to the present book was to look at the ways in which genetic knowledge gears itself to different kinds of social experience and vice versa. In a way, our purpose could be defined as an attempt to provide an anthropological perspective upon the relationship between different forms of knowledge. No general conclusion can be drawn, or should be drawn, from the rich and heterogeneous diversity of perspectives that this research has given rise to. More appropriately, this concluding chapter should be considered as a theoretical epilogue of sorts. I wish to analyse the conditions under which different forms of knowledge produce different forms of truth and meaning and, specifically, how these different forms interact with each other.

When bioethicists talk about the 'social character' of genetic information (e.g. Wert et al. 2003: 2), they do not mean that it is socially produced information, for all scientific information is. The social character of genetic information refers to its relational quality. Unlike any other kind of biomedical knowledge, its subject is not the individual but a group of interrelated individuals. This is going to be the central concern of this concluding chapter. Of all the social effects, social meanings, social character and social repercussions that genetic knowledge has or is likely to have, I wish to concentrate on only one particular aspect: genetic knowledge is knowledge about human relations, about the way humans are related to each other.[1]

Now the question is, given its relational character, will genetics change the way we understand human society? Will genetic knowledge change our social life, will it create new forms of social bonds, of 'biosociality' in Rabinow's terms (1996: 99), while it obliterates other forms?

Genetic knowledge is knowledge about genes, which in turn could be defined as DNA sequences that fulfil a particular function within the cell. The remarkable thing about genes is that in their combination they make each individual living organism, with the exception of identical twins, unique, different from any other organism that exists, has existed and will exist. Thus the uniqueness of each individual in genetic terms has nothing to do with its substance, but with the specific combination of its components, which are shared with all the other individual organisms. Biodiversity originates in the endless combinations and recombinations of a finite number of elements. '[T]he fact that everyone is part of someone else is held to conserve the individuality of each recombination' (Strathern 2005: 28). Since the genetic individuality of each human being lies in the specific and random combination of his or her parental DNA sequences, this can be defined as a *relational* individuality (see Porqueres i Gené and Wilgaux, this volume). Thus, even though genetic knowledge can be ideologically used to foster non-relational forms of individuality, the truth of the matter is that, from a strictly scientific point of view, the genetic individuality of each human being contains a statement about the relations between different individuals. Now these are first and foremost biogenetic relations: they consist of sharing genes. But they might be more than that, since in all human societies the reproduction of human beings through sexual intercourse is a socially regulated activity. Therefore, what for non-human living organisms is a mere sharing of DNA sequences, the object of knowledge of a scientific discipline such as molecular biology, for human beings it might involve the constitution of specific social relationships, the object of a form of social knowledge that we normally call kinship (see Porqueres i Gené 2004: 143–44). In what follows, I want to look at the ways in which we can relate knowledge of this particular kind of social relationship with knowledge of biogenetic connections and, more crucially perhaps, at the 'knowledge coalitions' (Rapp et al. 2001: 401) that might emerge from their interaction and reciprocal constitution.

But now it is the concept of relational individuality in strictly biogenetic terms that I wish to bring into focus. An individual's genotype has no specific substance other than sets of DNA sequences that he or she shares with his or her ancestors and descendants and with the individuals equally descendent from those ancestors and so on. Interestingly, what molecular biologists understand by 'gene sharing' is quite distinct from what seems to be implied, literally speaking at least, in notions of 'consanguinity' or 'consubstantiality'. From that perspective, there is no physical connection between an individual and his or her progenitors: that individual's DNA molecules do not come from them. To share genes does not mean to share any natural substance but to share information, 'intangible, non-material information' (Silver 2001: 652).[2]

Silver puts forward the analogy of computer files. There is no physical connection between all the copies of a file I can make in different computer discs, no matter is shared between them but only information, i.e. a pattern for organising matter (ibid. 652–53). The notion of blood as a programmer (Porqueres i Gené and Wilgaux, this volume) or Gypsies' conceptions of semen as a gas or a breath (Manrique, this volume) ought to be mentioned here. Conversely, when we look at what some anthropologists have found out in the field of kinship, for instance, Malay conceptions of relatedness as depicted by Carsten (1997), which happen to be not so distant from the way northern English mothers relate to their children, as analysed by Degnen (this volume), we see that kinship is understood in these contexts as resulting from food sharing rather than from consanguinity originating in sexual reproduction. From the point of view of molecular biology, following Silver's account (see note 2), both the Malay kinship concept and northern English understandings of motherhood would be closer to a biochemical definition of consubstantiality than conventional Euro-American definitions.

Forms of Knowledge and Forms of Truth

We have just seen that the idea of consubstantiality seems to be at odds with the nature of genetic relatedness according to scientific narratives. But the definition of kinship as a relation of consubstantiality is, at best, a rather simplistic one. I have argued that the relational nature of genetic knowledge is bound to have social meanings as regards human beings if only because reproduction through sexual intercourse, the origin of genetic relatedness, is a socially regulated activity in all human societies. But this is a much more controversial statement than appears at first sight. Ever since the beginnings of anthropological research, it has been observed that the universal or quasi-universal social regulation of sexual reproductive activity does not give rise to a structure of social relations coextensive with biogenetic pedigrees. Now how this lack of correspondence between kinship systems and biogenetic relations should be accounted for is a bone of contention in social anthropology. Following Durkheim, British anthropologists have traditionally seen kinship as a social construct with no necessary relation to the natural facts of human reproduction. But the social constructionist approach to the study of kinship systems presented two important theoretical dilemmas. First, a great deal of anthropological kinship theory has been developed on the assumption that kinship was universal, and the universality of kinship was predicated on its biological substrate, on the fact that it had to do with, it originated in, the 'facts of life': procreation, biological reproduction, etc. But if this biological substrate is no longer decisive in the definition of kinship, on what grounds are we going to defend its universality now? Secondly, if kinship is a 'pure' social relationship, it is unclear how are we going to differentiate it from other social relationships.

Implicitly or explicitly, theoretical debates in the anthropology of kinship have often been centred around the concepts of 'nature' and 'culture', their mutual interrelations and the forms of knowledge that presumably give access to them. Kinship is a form of social knowledge: it is knowledge about social relations. Human genetics is scientific knowledge, expert knowledge about natural entities produced by scientists in laboratories. But what do genes have to do with social life? How can a specialised and somewhat exclusive cognitive product such as genetics be engaged in the everyday experience of ordinary people?

In his analysis of lay beliefs about genetic inheritance in England, Richards (1997) found out that most people coming from families with hereditary diseases are not able to furnish an accurate account of Mendelian genetics, despite the fact that they are very interested in inheritance, have several beliefs and theories about it and have undoubtedly learnt about the science of genetics from genetic counselling and as part of their science curriculum when they were at school. 'What does seem possible is that some people who have received genetic counselling may see the inheritance of the specific condition that was the subject of the counselling in Mendelian terms, but their more general notion of inheritance may remain unaltered as a separate domain' (Richards 1997: 191). This separate domain is constituted by the kinship culture, Richards concludes, and, no matter how much knowledge of scientific theories on genetics is taught at schools or through genetic counselling, beliefs coming from the kinship culture seem to remain unaltered (see Darr 1997: 87; Davison 1997: 172–73). Does this mean that kinship and genetics are totally incommensurable forms of truth, that interactions and intersections between the two are impossible? As Čepaitienė has argued in this volume, 'participation in the constitution of the child as well as sharing of physicality and bodily links is not separable from the whole package of feelings, experiences, thoughts, events, relations – the "materialities" that compose and process the persons and their entire universes'.

From the scientists' perspective, it is customarily assumed that expert knowledge on human life produced by the biosciences should, and eventually will, flow downwards to meet the lay public demand for truth. This is what has been called above the 'deficit model' of public understanding of science (Edwards n.d.). This model is akin to what in the history of anthropological thought constituted the intellectualist view on so-called 'primitive' beliefs. The difference between 'us' and 'them', scientists and non-scientists, is merely the difference between those who possess truth knowledge and those who don't. 'Progress' means simply knowledge transfer from one pole to the other, from civilised to primitive, from scientists to lay public. But intellectualist perspectives have been long outdated in anthropology, in the same way as the deficit model has been forcefully criticised within the discipline of social studies of science (see Nowotny et al. 2001). Thus, 'what may be termed public understanding of the new genetics are not passive reflections of professional, scientific understandings; rather, they are active constructs, the products of multiply-mediated historical and cultural (including the media) influences' (Durant et al. 1996: 236).

As anthropologists we can see that this model of knowledge transfer is seriously misleading on several counts. On the one hand, it is based on the assumption of an uncontested truth monopoly enjoyed by expert scientific knowledge in Western societies. On the other, and more importantly, it takes for granted that the 'will to truth', paradigmatic of modern scientific activity, will play in ordinary people's lives the same prominent role as in the scientists' practice. But, once we abandon the deficit model of knowledge, the idea that scientific truth knowledge merely flows unilaterally and unmediated from scientists to non-scientists, the question we should try to answer is how the spread of scientific knowledge is likely to affect lay cognitive systems, in other words, how scientific knowledge is going to be translated into culturally meaningful knowledge.

Cadoret uses in this volume a recently published text by Foucault (2003) directly relevant to our purposes. 'A knowledge such as the one we call science', Foucault contends, 'is a knowledge that supposes, in reality, that there is a truth everywhere and at all times' (my translation, Foucault 2003: 235). Scientific truth is a non-personal, universal, truth. Foucault defines it in different ways: *'vérité connaissance'*, *'vérité de démonstration'*, *'vérité découverte'*, *'vérité constatation'*, *'vérité apophantique'*, etc. (2003: 237–38). This form of truth is not restricted to the scientific mode of knowledge, although it seems that in modern science it has reached its paramount development. And scientific truth is nowhere to be found but in nature, in the reality of the natural world and natural entities; hence the need for scientists, since the beginnings of the scientific revolution in the seventeenth century, to carry out experiments in order to prove the veracity of their statements (Shapin 1996: 69). 'Since the Enlightenment, Western culture has trained us to look for scientific truth in every natural fact' (Cadoret, this volume). For scientists nature is the sole source of truth and knowledge, and the truth of nature exists by itself, even if humans ignore it. As I have pointed out, this form of truth is not the exclusive domain of science, but the fact that in science it has been endowed with primordial value, the fact that it has been carried out to its last consequences by all available means and with a widely recognised efficacy, deeply affects other non-scientific forms of knowledge equally concerned with the same or very similar forms of truth.

But in the history of Western civilisation, Foucault goes on, there is also another kind of truth, different from scientific truth. This is a 'dispersed, discontinued, interrupted' truth. It comes only from certain subjects, from certain places, it is an 'event truth' (*vérité-événement*). Between the event truth and its object there is not a relationship of knowledge (*rapport de connaissance*), as is the case with discovered truth, there is a relationship of power (Foucault 2003: 236–37). An instance of this event truth can be found in the judicial processes of the Middle Ages. Torture was systematically used in them to make the suspect tell the 'truth'. But what kind of truth was that? Torture was not a way to obtain a demonstrative truth, as in modern judicial process, but was a 'physical struggle' between the judges and the suspect. The suspect's confession was a sign that he had lost the struggle: thus he could be condemned. Foucault also calls this form of truth *'vérité-rapport du pouvoir'* or simply *'vérité-rituel'*, ritual truth (2003: 238).

Drawing inspiration from Lévi-Strauss's (1962) renowned analysis, I would like to transform Foucault's distinction into a theory of forms of knowledge. There is one form of knowledge concerned with establishing cause-and-effect links between phenomena, syntagmatic relations. I shall call this type of knowledge truth knowledge, the knowledge that produces 'truth'. But there is also a second type, which, in contrast, aims at producing meanings through paradigmatic connections. Let us call it symbolic knowledge. Obviously, by these terms it is not being suggested that truth knowledge is meaningless, any more than symbolic knowledge is false. In a sense, it could be argued that both kinds of knowledge are equally true and meaningful. But the relationship between truth and meaning are the opposite in one and the other. The meaning of truth knowledge is the search for truth, the accurate representation of the real – demonstrative truth, in Foucault's terms. The truth of symbolic knowledge is the search for meaning, i.e. the constitution of significant cultural values and beliefs for a particular community – ritual truth.

We should keep in mind that symbolic knowledge is social knowledge, it gains its legitimacy – its 'truth', if you like – from a particular set of social relationships, it is inherent to the very nature of those social relationships. The truth about filiation, argues Cadoret in this volume, 'is not a universal truth, independent of the actual members in the family, but true only when applied to particular families, a particular family constellation'. Manrique's definition of truth as 'shared experiences of life' (this volume) could also be seen as another instance of it. Truth knowledge, in contrast, is individual, asocial, knowledge in the sense that it gains its legitimacy not from the value it confers upon a set of social relationships but from its accuracy and precision as a representation of the real world (what Foucault would call *'rapport de connaissance'*). An instance of this form of knowledge can be found in this volume in Campbell's analysis of the media's treatment of GMO. Campbell contends that 'Ecological science was imagined to speak for itself, or to stand as a view on what was happening "out there", with the issue of people's relationship to the landscape silently contained' (Campbell, this volume).

An important caveat should be entered now. To define truth knowledge as 'asocial' knowledge does not mean in any conceivable way that it is not socially produced. This is not an analytical assertion concerning the way knowledge is produced in human societies or by human individuals but merely a descriptive ethnographic statement of the emic forms of legitimacy of different forms of knowledge. In other words, I am not trying to answer the theoretical question 'What is science' but the ethnographic one 'What do people think when they think about science?' If we take science as an outstanding example of truth knowledge, what I am arguing is simply that the social determinants of scientific statements do not figure among their truth conditions, i.e. the conditions that confer validity to those statements within the scientific community. I hope that the ensuing examples of truth knowledge will help to clarify this point.

Be this as it may, the remarkable fact about forms of knowledge is that they do not thrive in isolation but in constant interrelation and intersection. And here is where we shall concentrate our attention now. We shall be looking at the two forms of knowledge of human relatedness that we call genetics and kinship, on the assumption that genetics is about truth knowledge and kinship about symbolic knowledge.[3] As has been stated, it could be surmised that truth knowledge should figure prominently in science, genetics in our case, whereas symbolic knowledge ought to predominate in non-scientific cognitive systems, namely kinship. But this is no more than an a priori judgement.

Uncertain Motherhood

There are contexts that have nothing to do either with scientific research or with medical reasons in which an explicit will to know arises, originating in a need for a naked, 'meaningless', truth that does not seem to play any role in the constitution of kinship or any other significant social relationship, a pure *'rapport de connaissance'*. Let me illustrate this will to know with a vignette from the ethnographic research I have been carrying out in western Ireland, intermittently, since the early 1990s. In the summer of 2002, an old friend of mine took me to a cemetery to show me his mother's tomb. My friend had been a foster-child in one of the local farms, so it was his foster-mother's tomb we were going to see. He was a foster-child but he knew who his birth mother was. Some time before we met he had begun to search for her. He discovered then that, like many other foster- and adopted children in rural Ireland, he had been a foster-child because he had been conceived out of wedlock. In those days (about fifty years ago), illegitimacy was a grave sin in rural Ireland. Unmarried mothers were heavily censured and suffered from ostracism within their communities (Salazar 2006: 43ff.). While my friend's birth mother was pregnant, she met a man who agreed to marry her on condition that she should get rid of the child as soon as he or she was born. The child went to a home and was eventually fostered by a farming family (see Salazar 1999).

After meeting his birth mother for the first time in his life, the two of them entertained for a while an amicable relationship, which suddenly came to an end some months later. Disagreements cropped up between my friend and his birth mother for all sorts of different reasons. She was trying to tell him how he should bring up his children, and wanted to interfere in his relationship with his wife. None of that was her business, he explained. Apparently, it was my friend who actually broke up the relationship himself. At no time did he manifest any regrets for what he had done, nor did he seem to be very interested in resuming the contact with his birth mother. In view of his rather cool and indifferent attitude, I asked him why he had searched for his birth mother in the first place. He answered very convincingly that it had been because of his eldest son. Once the son asked him for his grandmother: 'Who is my granny, dad?' Confronted with this very simple question my friend realised that he had no answer for it, so he decided to begin his search. It was just a matter of curiosity more than anything else, he commented.

It is clear from this that for my informant the blood relation that linked him to his birth mother did not seem to be particularly meaningful. Was it the need for truth knowledge and not the need for social bonds that impelled him to look for her? I think there was a bit of both actually, especially taking into account the rather ambivalent relationship that he always kept with his foster-mother when she was alive. Besides, what triggered off my friend's search was his son's 'kinship' question – who is my granny? (But was that really a 'kinship' question?) Whatever it was, he was telling me all that while we were approaching the cemetery. The cemetery was on top of a hill, close to an ancient holy well, a very common burial ground in some parishes of western Ireland. Now there is a little road that takes you just in front of the gates. But this is only recent; when the mother died (remember, the foster-mother), only a few years ago, you could only reach the cemetery by going across the fields. And yet the mother insisted that she wanted to be buried in that graveyard. Why? Because there her blood relatives had been buried, her own mother and her two sons, who died of pneumonia while they were very young. My friend emphasised the significance of having her blood relations in that cemetery as the only thing that could explain why she insisted so much on being buried there herself, despite the obvious difficulties involved in carrying the coffin across the fields when there was no road. While we were in front of the old woman's tomb, my friend said a short prayer while his eyes were filling with tears: a natural reaction, perhaps, for someone in front of his or her mother's grave.

Before we left he told me a bit about the different people and their relatives who had been buried in that cemetery. I asked him then if he wished to be buried there himself. No, he did not. 'This is not my place,' he explained.

I wanted to draw the reader's attention to the complex and paradoxical way in which both the meaningfulness and the meaninglessness of kinship, on the one hand, and biogenetic relations, on the other, are thrown into relief in this brief ethnographic snapshot. Clearly, I believe, if my informant recognised any bond that we might identify as 'kinship' it was with his foster-mother, not with his birth mother. With care, we can interpret his search for his birth mother as an attempt to get truth knowledge, to get at a demonstrative truth devoid of any social meaning.

'People want to know which box they slot into,' one of Edwards's informants asserted while comparing adoption with the anonymity of gamete donation in assisted reproduction (Edwards 1993: 61). An analogous need to know one's roots seems to be at the root of the 'motherland tours' organised by Norwegian transnational adoptive parents with their adoptive children, according to Howell's account (2003). None of the adoptive children who go on these tours have any interest in meeting their blood relatives, let alone in setting up any kind of bond with them. In fact, Howell surmises that the purpose of the motherland tours is more to confirm the adoptees' Norwegianness than to embrace their origins. And yet the need to know one's (biological) origins seems to be taken for granted. So much so that the Norwegian parliament has decided to rescind anonymity in sperm donation on the assumption that, in the words of the Minister for Children and Families, 'knowledge of biological origin has enormous emotional significance for individual persons' (cited in Melhuus 2003: 183). In a similar vein, Carsten has argued in her analysis of adoption reunions in Britain that they have nothing to do with the search for one's blood or 'real' relatives. Rather, they should be interpreted as a way to recover a sense of agency over one's own past (Carsten 2000b: 689): with 'recovering a lost biography, with becoming a complete person, and with the desire to fill in the gaps' (2000b: 694). In a revealing example, Carsten (2004: 103–151) cites the case of a woman whose birth father insisted on denying his paternity. But she managed to prove it, thanks to DNA screening of a half-brother on her father's side. Clearly, the woman did not have any interest in using DNA testing to establish a bond with that man, she just wanted to 'stop the lies' and 'waft the results under his nose' (Carsten 2004: 104); in other words, she wanted to 'establish the truth' (2004: 151; see also Nelkin and Lindee 1995: 66–72; Dooley et al. 2003: 45; Konrad 2003). The same could be said concerning the way some adoptive parents justify their preference for open adoptions: according to Marre and Bestard (this volume), they wish to know their child's biological parents but they do not want to establish any relation with them. In Norway, the revelation of King Olav's dubious conception generated some interest in the media, but the legitimacy of the monarchy was not questioned, and, in a similar way, the abolition of the anonymity clause in sperm donation does not confer filiation rights on the sperm donor (Melhuus and Howell, this volume).

In all these examples, we could say that the 'will to know' biogenetic connections does not seem to form the substrate of any meaningful social bond. It is as if a geneticist or genetic counsellor told us from whom we inherited a particular gene: he also has no interest in reinforcing or weakening the bond that we might have with that particular person. The geneticist only wants us to know an impersonal and universal truth – even though the lay interlocutor's response to this impersonal truth may range from its acceptance as a sort of 'revelation' of one's true being to different forms of objection or utter refusal (Rapp 1999: 165ff.).

But this is only half of the story. Let us get back for a minute to the case from the west of Ireland mentioned above. My informant did not see any bond in the truth that led him to his birth mother, and yet at the same time he did not underestimate the significance of blood or biogenetic links, both in the way he empathetically described his mother's desire to be buried with her blood relatives, her own mother and her two children, despite the difficulties entailed in such an endeavour, and also in the way in which he manifested his desire not be buried there (when those difficulties, incidentally, have disappeared because of the new road). The question is now: where do we find 'more' kinship? In my friend's relationship with his foster-mother or in the relationship of his foster-mother with her blood relatives buried in that cemetery? Undoubtedly, kinship is in both places, although 'genes', biogenetic links, exist only in one of them.

An oscillation between biologised and de-biologised or geneticised and de-geneticised conceptions of relatedness has been recurrently observed in different situations. Čepaitienė points out in this volume that some of her informants 'see the sperm donor like a "stranger (*svetimas*)" in the family who through the act of donation "has sex" with the inseminated woman, brings with him his juridical rights to the child and his "genetic tree" – that is kinship'. Similarly, the woman who was about to have an IVF with egg donation in Bestard's account (this volume) manifested her fear that some day the father might argue that since the child was genetically his he could take him or her away from the mother. But, in a totally different situation, the Catalan adopted girl who went to meet her Indian biological parents (Marre and Bestard, this volume) claimed that 'it is my people without it really being my people, because there is nothing apart from the physical aspect that joins us'. In transnational adoptions in Norway, on the other hand, Howell (2001: 206) has seen how 'in some contexts ... biological explanatory models are foregrounded at the expense of sociocultural ones, and in other contexts, sociocultural models are foregrounded while those of biology are ignored'. The same was observed by Ragoné (1994: 137) among participants in surrogacy arrangements, that they 'pick and choose among American cultural values about family, parenthood, and reproduction, now choosing biological relatedness, now nurture, as it suits their needs', and by Cadoret (2003, this volume) among French homosexual couples who wish to have children either by adoption or by assisted conception, that they also tend to alternate between biological and non-biological definitions of parenthood.

Now, for a better understanding of this ambivalent, oscillating and sometimes plainly contradictory meaning with which biogenetic connections seem to be endowed, I wish to show a second ethnographic vignette. This time it comes from the research conducted by my colleague Gemma Orobitg among egg donors in an infertility clinic in Barcelona (see

Orobitg and Salazar 2005). Several women who had donated their eggs or who were about to do so were interviewed. Orobitg realised that, in addition to annoying physical hardships, these women were also going through a number of ethical and cognitive dilemmas in order to make sense of their act. Egg donors tended to define their behaviour in ethical terms. Their action was understood as a form of help towards another woman, as the enactment of a moral duty to help other women. Whatever the particular significance that the economic compensation they received could have (800 euros), they very rarely foregrounded economic reasons as an explanation for egg donation. The overall moral value of their action, however, was clearly insufficient to render their behaviour fully meaningful in cognitive terms. Very often they compared egg donation with blood donation: you donate something, part of your body, to help someone else. It is the same, really, but it is different as well. But what is the difference? Is it because you are actually donating your genes?

In the interviews, my colleague tried to find out what was the meaning of genes, of genetic links, for these women. Quite obviously, perhaps, none of them considered that the genes they were donating would create any bond. They recognised that the child born from their eggs might 'take after them'; he or she will have 'something from them'. But by no means could that be seen as kinship. The mother is the one who will give birth after nine months of pregnancy, the one who will bring the child up and will look after him/her with love and affection. They, egg donors, only provide the means, so to speak, for a woman to do that. One woman even talked of genes in disparaging terms: 'The child will have some of my genes, that's all,' she said, clearly implying that genes in themselves were totally or nearly meaningless (see Konrad 1998: 651–52). We are reminded here of the Hungarian foster-mothers studied by Demény in this volume, who emphasised gene sharing while thinking about how important it might be for men to have their own children, whereas for women biological motherhood was defined in terms of pregnancy and birth but not by the sharing of genes.

In any case, these were perfectly natural and foreseeable reactions for women in those particular conditions. They had no interest in looking at motherhood in genetic terms, so they decided to define kinship in a different way. They decided to think about motherhood in such a way that genetic links did not seem to play any role. Genes fell into the background, even further away, while other aspects of the kinship relationship were foregrounded: love, affection, day-to-day contact, even clearly biological aspects such as pregnancy and parturition. So, if genes did not seem to make any difference, what could be the difference between egg donation and blood donation – or any other form of organ donation for that matter? None of the interviewed women could formulate in precise terms what was so specific to egg donation.[4] But, from the conversations Orobitg had with them, it was clear that the connection with motherhood had something to do with it: not, or not only, in the obvious sense that it was a way of helping another woman to have a child, to become a mother, but also because several women saw egg donation as a form of ancillary motherhood, an almost 'metonymic' motherhood.

Two of the interviewees had had previous abortions. One of them did not want to talk about it, but the other explained that, for her, egg donation was a way of compensating for the effects of that dreadful experience. In tears, she told the researcher that she was very young at that time, she did not want to do it but it had been because of family pressures that she decided to take that course of action. She had been suffering from a kind of remorse ever since. There was something very deep inside her that she could not get rid of, no matter what. By helping another woman to become a mother she was hoping to somehow attenuate her guilty feelings. In a much less emotional tone, another woman, who already had two children and who for medical and financial reasons could have no more, said quite openly that she saw egg donation as a 'different way of being a mother', even though, she added immediately, it won't be a child of her own.

Certainly, none of these women considered themselves to be the 'real' mothers of their genetic children, the children that would eventually be born thanks to their donation. But at the same time it could not be denied that by donating their eggs a sort of symbolic motherhood came into existence: a symbolic motherhood that would somehow make up for the lost motherhood because of an abortion, or similarly it might substitute for the desired motherhood that for different reasons could not be achieved. Egg donation was for these women a metonymy for motherhood, the symbolic substitute for something non-existent but deeply longed for. It is instructive to compare this symbolic motherhood with the symbolic (biological) relatedness that adoptive parents establish with their children who 'resemble' them, following Marre and Bestard's study (this volume): in the one case a real biological bond symbolises an non-existent social relationship, whereas in the other it is an non-existent biological bond that symbolises a real social relationship. Still, whether the genetic bond that links these symbolic mothers to their children-to-be plays any significant role in the constitution of this relationship cannot be fully ascertained.[5]

Bodies and substances in people's narration stand not for themselves, but for persons (Čepaitienė, this volume). Be that as it may, my wish is to remark on the paradox entailed in denying real motherhood, on the one hand, and imagining symbolic motherhood, on the other. Remember that this is very similar to the paradoxical attitude that we saw in my Irish informant, simultaneously emphasising and underestimating the significance of blood ties.

Intersections

What can we learn from these two bits of ethnography concerning the relationships between genetics and kinship, between the truth knowledge of genetics and the symbolic knowledge of kinship? A first and rather obvious point, which nevertheless needs to be recalled, is that the symbolic knowledge of kinship is a culturally constructed form of knowledge. Thus, for genetic knowledge to be relevant in a particular kinship system, genes must have cultural value, that is, they must be meaningful in terms of the kinship system (and not merely 'true' in biological terms). Consider the situation of the egg donors. Whatever the truth value that genetic science may attribute to that what links them to their genetic children (the children to be born from their eggs), for them this gene sharing is meaningless, or nearly meaningless. To emphasise this meaninglessness, they draw on different tropes that equally define motherhood but take no consideration of genetic links: love, affection, parturition, etc. Whatever new truths genetic science might produce concerning genes and their properties, there is no doubt that they will have very little repercussion upon the meanings that kinship and motherhood have for these women. Still, it is unclear whether genes have no value at all in cultural terms since, as we have seen, they might constitute the signifier of another kinship tie of sorts.[6]

Consider now the case from western Ireland. Blood relations (note that these are not necessarily genetic relations, but we can leave that aside since it does not affect my main point) are culturally relevant in the west of Ireland, as exemplified by my friend's mother's desire to be buried with her blood relatives, or his own desire not to be buried there himself. And yet this cultural value did not prevent him from considering as his mother his foster-mother instead of his birth mother, or at least from feeling more emotionally attached to the first woman than to the second. Again, what we can see here is a creative use of the cultural values that configure a particular kinship system. Both situations throw into relief the fact that the translation of truth knowledge into symbolic knowledge is a complex one. It is complex because the second type of knowledge depends for its validation on a particular set of social relationships. 'The "truth" of kinship cannot be solved by reference to biology, as in our society we used to think' (Bestard 2004a: 262). In a somewhat aphoristic fashion, it could be said that the meaning of genes for a kinship system is not contingent upon their truth – something that clearly calls into question Schneider's view of kinship as whatever science says it is. The virtue of genetic discourses is not so much their novelty but rather 'their capacity to bring people back *to what they already know*' (Strathern 2005: 30). But how is that possible?

That cultural meanings are systematically related in such a way that they depend on each other for their validation, and not on the 'real' objects they presumably refer to, constitutes one of the most elementary principles of the structural theory of language and culture (see Bestard, this volume). I wish to see the validity of this time-honoured approach in my analysis of the intersections between genetics and kinship. When we ask ourselves whether genetic knowledge will be relevant in a particular social context such as a kinship system, we are actually wondering about the capacity of genes to signify, and to be signified by, cultural values. This is a question that strikes deeply into the heart of anthropological debates on kinship theory. For years anthropologists have been discussing what sort of relation could be established between the genealogical grid of a kinship system – that is, the ramifying chain of culturally constructed parent-child links and marital ties, as Goodenough (2001: 207) has defined it – and biogenetic pedigrees. I believe that the time-honoured definition of kinship as the mere attribution of particular social functions to biological ties between individuals is inadequate because the existence of these biological ties, a truth knowledge, does not necessarily mean that they have to be socially significant in any way. Atoms and molecules have existed for hundreds of millions of years and yet the majority of human societies did not confer any particular meaning upon them. But it would be equally wrong to conceive that the relationship between the genealogical grid of a kinship system and biogenetic pedigrees is merely contingent or, even worse, that biogenetic pedigrees cannot be held to exist unless they have been culturally recognised by a particular kinship system in the first place. Such an unseemly conclusion is the result of a confusion between truth knowledge and symbolic knowledge. The fact that we human individuals share part of our genetic make-up is a consequence of the way in which our species is biologically reproduced. This statement is biological truth knowledge that does not depend for its legitimacy on its cultural recognition by any kinship system, or by any other socially constructed set of cultural values for that matter. In the same way as atoms and molecules existed for millions of years even if humans did not know anything about them, human beings (like any other living organism) share part of their genetic endowments even if no social function or cultural meaning is attributed to such a fact.

When science discovers new facts about genes there is no need for any kinship system to ascertain the truth of such discoveries. Scientific knowledge is, as I said before, asocial knowledge, it gains its legitimacy, its truth value, not from culture or social relations but from its capacity to constitute itself as an accurate representation of the real world. But scientific discoveries in genetics do not automatically translate themselves into cultural meanings: we need a kinship system to do this job. But how? How can kinship translate truth into meaning? This is not a trivial question because there is nothing in the concept of kinship (the ramifying chain of culturally constructed parent-child links and marital ties) that calls for the scientific knowledge of genetic matter for its validation. This might sound a bit counter-intuitive, taking into account that our word for genealogy is cognate with our word for gene. But this is a mere lexical red herring: kinship systems have existed for thousands of years in a myriad of different societies with no knowledge of genetics and obviously with no word for gene (or indeed genealogy) or anything remotely resembling it.

In their analysis of the symbolic meaning of the word gene in so-called 'popular culture', Nelkin and Lindee (1995: 16) maintain that a gene is not a biological entity. 'Though it refers to a biological construct and derives its cultural power from science, its symbolic meaning is independent of biological definitions.' In a similar vein, French biologist Jean Pierre Changeux (2003: 9) has stated that, 'out of its scientific context, turned into a "social representation" and put at the service of politics and the media, the symbolic meaning of the word gene or even of genetics has been diverted from its object' (my translation). I believe that the kinship system has played a crucial role in the emergence of the symbolic power of genes. 'Kinship is not only a system of meaning that uses facts of nature to signify social relations; it is also a tool of translation between nature and culture' (Bestard 2004a: 260). But perhaps the capacity of kinship to divert the concept of gene from its object, i.e. to translate genetic truth into cultural meaning, has nothing to do with its substance (parent-child links and marital ties), no matter how counter-intuitive this might sound to us at first blow, but it is to do with its form. We have already seen that substantivist definitions of kinship, such as sharing blood, flesh, biological matter, etc., are clearly at odds with scientific notions of genetic relatedness. Even the idea of 'sharing genes', separated from its proper scientific context, as Changeux would say, is likely to be scientifically inadequate, for genes are shared between all living organisms but we do not consider all living organisms as 'kin'. But what about if we see kinship as a form instead of as a substance?

Formal analyses in the anthropology of kinship were fashionable in the 1950s and 1960s, especially in the USA. They were based on the principle that genealogical relations were universal, so that all kinship systems – by which they meant kinship terminological systems – could be translated, quite often through complex algebraic operations, into genealogical types. That is what formal analyses of kinship systems were all about. Critics argued that the principle of the universality of the genealogical grid was unwarranted. There was no a priori reason to believe that genealogical relations, based as they were on the 'givens' of biological reproduction, should receive cultural significance the world over; only ethnography can tell what is and what is not culturally significant in any one particular society. But some current formalist approaches seem to be on the verge of overcoming that traditional objection. Their strategy is apparently to push kinship analysis further up in the scale of abstraction so that any 'substantivist' vestige, such as the belief in the universality of the givens of biological reproduction, can be conveniently removed. How do we define kinship then from this perspective? 'Kinship is a system of interrelated definitions of a set of interrelated social positions' (Leaf 2001: 70). It is no longer a question of translating kin terms into genealogical kin types but merely into a set of interrelated positions in a logical space with its own internal consistency and with no reference to any external 'substantive' object, be this biology, genealogy, biogenetic pedigrees or whatever it may be. Some will certainly dislike this definition for being too abstract, too remote from ordinary understandings of kinship and, more critically perhaps, too broad to allow us to differentiate kinship from other kinds of social relatedness. Be that as it may, the interesting thing about this approach is that it turns the kinship system into the potential signifier both of the genealogical grid and, alternatively or simultaneously, of the social positions that may be in structural correspondence to it. According to Read (2001: 81), a talented advocate of this approach, the 'linkage between the terminological space and a genealogical grid is elucidated by analytically mapping the terminological space onto the genealogical grid. The mapping, then, determines for each of the abstract symbols in the terminological structure its definition as a class of associated kin types.' But the terminological space can be equally mapped onto 'a collection of persons without necessarily making reference to genealogical claims' (Read 2001: 100; see also McKinley 2001: 158–60). In other words, at a sufficient level of abstraction, we can turn the kinship system, understood as a logically consistent and autonomous terminological space, into the symbol of any external system that can be 'mapped onto' it, be this the genealogical grid, a social structure or, a fortiori, a biogenetic pedigree. 'If this is true, nether nature nor culture is essentialised, but rather they become metaphors for thinking and imagining relatedness' (Bestard, this volume).

The symbolic power of genes is losing its aura of mystery. 'The cultural understanding ... of a scientific entity does not come from its contents, but from the relations that can be established with other heterogeneous materialities' (my translation, Bestard 2003: 234). Genes can signify, and be signified by, the cultural values of a kinship system, that is, the 'substance' of a kinship system, because of the structural correspondence or homology between the form of a genetic pedigree and the form of the kinship system. This means that the substance of kinship has no biogenetic content, even though it might have it in specific circumstances, in specific speech acts, so to say, because of the homology between the form of kinship and the form of biogenetic pedigrees. Conversely, we could say that the substance of genetics has no social content, even though it might have it in specific circumstances because of the same reason, the formal homology between kinship and biogenetic relations.[7] Furthermore, in so far as biogenetic links connect humans with non-human living organisms in a syntagmatic chain, as Campbell has contended in his provocative contribution to this volume, the structural homology between kinship and genes finds its limit in the substantive analogy between all living beings. Hence genes become a metaphor for human social relationships and a metonymy for the relationships between humans and non-human beings.

Godelier (2004: 340) has recently argued that the relationship between kinship and society can be expressed in terms of a double metamorphosis. Social forms that have nothing to do with kinship, such as landownership, political relations, etc., 'lodge themselves' into a kinship structure and put it at their service while, at the same time, those social forms transform themselves into aspects of that kinship structure (see Salazar 2004). In a similar vein, we could claim that biogenetic relations constitute a further dimension of this double metamorphosis. Genes can put a kinship structure at their service in such as way that they can be symbolised or referred to by a kinship language while at the same time they transform themselves into aspects of a kinship bond. But, similarly to landownership and political relations, genes can be symbols because they are not substances but relational entities. It is the relational nature of genetic knowledge that turns it into a potential signifier or signified of cultural meanings equally relational, such as the kinship system. It is the relational nature of kinship knowledge that turns it into 'a potent combination with which to imagine relations of all kinds, not just the family kind' (Edwards 2000: 27). Now, as for the content of these symbols, that is what we, lay people, scientists, geneticists, medical doctors, mean when we talk about genes, about our relatives, about genes and relatives, about relatives who share genes and relatives who don't, about sets of moral values, beliefs, theories about the person, about rights and obligations, about identity and difference, etc., all this can only be elucidated through ethnographic research. My purpose has been merely to expose the structural conditions that might account for the emergence of those symbols and their meanings.

Notes

1. In fact, genetic knowledge is about all living organisms, humans and non-humans, even though here I am only interested in its repercussions upon human relations.
2. 'And where did the DNA molecules in my body come from? They were actually built up, piece by piece, from smaller molecules that came from the cows, chickens, fish, plants and other things that my mother ate while she was pregnant, and that I have eaten since. The old saying 'you are what you eat' is not far from the truth in purely material terms.' (Silver 2001: 652)
3. Kaja Finkler's (2000) analysis on the medicalisation of kinship in American society brought about by the spread of genetic knowledge can be taken as a good instance of the intersection that concerns us here. Notably, Finkler's research suggests that the sort of truth knowledge that her informants wished to find out while searching for their biological relatives is not a monopoly of science. See Strathern's recent reassessment of the relationships between kinship and knowledge (2005: 67–75; see also Franklin 2003).
4. See Simpson (2004) for an interesting comparative reference to organ, blood and gamete donation in Sri Lanka.
5. Edwards's ethnography in north-west England has also captured this ambiguity in one of her informants' reflections on egg donation: 'Even though you haven't give birth to that child, it's been your eggs and it's born from your eggs, isn't it?' (2004: 762). It is clear from this ethnography, however, according to Edwards's interpretation, that motherhood in English kinship thinking, even in its more biologised sense, is never equivalent to the sharing of biogenetic substance. My feeling is that egg donors' symbolic motherhood might well originate in the sheer physicality of egg donation rather than in the actual genes that will be shared. Perhaps it is the metaphor of parturition, represented in the surgical removal of the eggs, rather than the metonymy of gene sharing, that constitutes this symbolic link.

6. What Strathern (2005: 76) has called relatedness without relatives but with signifying others.
7. In the ethnography above, my informant from Ireland could simultaneously disregard the biogenetic link that unites him to his birth mother and emphasise the importance of blood ties in the determination of particular burial places. Similarly, egg donors could deny or ignore the existence of any bond between themselves and their genetic children while at the same time they could imagine a symbolic motherhood stemming from their donation. Now the concept of motherhood that we should apply to make sense both of my Irish friend's attitude and that of egg donors cannot have any biogenetic content, otherwise we could understand neither the man's attachment to his foster-mother nor egg donors' denial of their kinship with their genetic children. But motherhood, a kinship concept, taken as a form, not as a substance, happens to be structurally homologous with the form that motherhood takes not as a kinship concept but as a biogenetic concept, that is, the female individual who has transferred half of her genetic endowment to another individual or individuals, to her offspring. That is the reason why the kinship concept of motherhood can also signify biogenetic motherhood and vice versa.

Notes on Contributors

Joan Bestard completed his doctorate in Social Anthropology at the University of Barcelona, where he is a senior lecturer and at present Head of the Department of Anthropology. He has carried out extensive ethnographic fieldwork in the Balearic Islands. He is interested in the social and cultural implications of new reproductive and genetic technologies. His latest publications include: 'Kinship and the New Genetics. The Changing Meaning of Biogenetic Substance', *Social Anthropology* (2004), *Parentesco y Reproducción Asistida: Cuerpo, Persona y Relaciones* (as co-author, Universidad de Barcelona, 2004), *Parentesco y Modernidad* (Barcelona: Paidós, 1998), and 'Memòria i continuïtat: el parentiu com a forma d'identitat', *Quaderns* (2000–2001).

Anne Cadoret is a senior researcher in Social Anthropology at the Centre National de la Recherche Scientifique, in Paris. She is studying plural families in France, and her main research has focused on fostering families and on homosexual parenthood. She is the author of *Parenté plurielle. Anthropologie du placement familial* (L'Harmattan, 1995) and *Des parents comme les autres. Homosexualité et parenté* (Odile Jacob, 2002).

Ben Campbell is Lecturer in Anthropology at the University of Durham, teaching previously at the universities of Edinburgh, Keele, Manchester and Hull. He has conducted fieldwork in the Nepal Himalayas on farming social practice, and environmental relationships in a Tibeto-Burman language community. He has published extensively on the cultural politics of indigenous knowledge and development, and environmental protection, and in 2005 edited the collection 'Re-placing Nature' in *Conservation and Society*.

Auksuolė Čepaitienė is a Senior Research Fellow in the Department of Ethnology, Lithuanian Institute of History, Vilnius. She has carried out research in various parts of Lithuania and in border areas in Belorussia and Poland, and has been interested in folk culture, social and cultural change and identity. She has published a book and various articles based on her previous studies. She has a special interest in local conceptions of ethnicity and kinship.

Cathrine Degnen is Lecturer in Social Anthropology at the University of Newcastle in the School of Geography, Politics and Sociology. She gained her MA and PhD at McGill University in Medical Anthropology and Anthropology, respectively, and was a postdoctoral researcher at the University of Manchester in Social Anthropology. In addition to her work on public understandings of genetics, she has research interests in experience and the self; ageing; social memory, place and temporality. Other recent and upcoming publications include articles in *The Sociological Review* and *The Journal of Aging Studies* and a chapter in *Creativity and Temporality* (Berg).

Enikő Demény is currently working as a researcher at the Central European University's Center for Ethics and Law in Biomedicine. She has a PhD in Philosophy, an MA in Cultural Anthropology and a BA in Sociology from the Babes-Bolyai University, Cluj, Romania, and an MA in Gender Studies from Central European University, Budapest. At present she is also a visiting lecturer at the Faculty of European Studies of Babes-Bolyai University, where she teaches courses on the MA programme on Anthropology and on Gender, Differences, Inequalities. She is a member of the Institute for Cultural Anthropology of Babes-Bolyai University.

Jeanette Edwards is Professor of Social Anthropology at Manchester University, UK. She has carried out extensive ethnographic fieldwork in the north of England and has published widely on kinship, new reproductive technologies and 'the public understanding of science'. She coordinated and directed the European-funded project 'Public Understanding of Genetics: a cross-cultural and ethnographic study of the "new genetics" and social identity' from which this volume stems.

Signe Howell is Professor of Social Anthropology at the University of Oslo. She has been undertaking research on transnational adoption in Norway and as a global phenomenon since 1999 and has published widely on the topic, including the book *The Kinning of Foreigners: Transnational Adoption in a Global Perspective* (Berghahn Books, 2006). Her previous research has been on religion, ritual and kinship in Malaysia and Indonesia.

Nathalie Manrique is completing her PhD in Social Anthropology at l'École des Hautes Études en Sciences Sociales in Paris about Gypsy representations of body and kinship in two small towns near Granada in southern Spain. She published 'La lune pétrifiée. Représentations parthénogénétiques dans une communauté gitane (Grenade)', in *Corps et Affects*, edited by Françoise Héritier and Margarita Xanthakou (Paris: Odile Jacob, 2004).

Diana Marre is a senior researcher at the Barcelona Centre of Childhood and the Urban World (CIIMU) and the University of Barcelona. She completed her doctorate in Social Anthropology at the University of Barcelona. Her publications include *La adopción y el acogimiento. Presente y perspectivas* (as co-editor, Universidad de Barcelona, 2004); 'To Kin a Foreign Child in Norway and Spain: Notions of Resemblances and the Achievement of Belonging' (as co-author, *Ethnos)*; and '"I Want she Learn her Language and Maintain her Culture": Transnational Adoptive Families' Views on "Cultural Origins"', in P. Wade (ed.) *Race, Ethnicity and Nation in Europe: Perspectives from Kinship and Genetics* (Berghahn Books, 2007).

Marit Melhuus, Professor of Social Anthropology at the University of Oslo, has done research in Argentina and Mexico and published extensively within economic anthropology, gender and morality, including a co-edited volume *Machos, Mistresses, Madonnas. Contesting the Power of Latin American Gender Imagery* (Verso, 1996). More recently she has been working in Norway addressing issues of kinship, biotechnology and law and has published several articles on these interlinked themes, with a specific focus on legislative processes and state formation. Tangentially she has addressed the theme of the transnational flow of concepts and substances and is co-editor of *Holding Worlds Together: Ethnographies of Knowing and Belonging* (Berghahn, 2007).

Enric Porqueres i Gené is Maître de Conférences at the Ecole des Hautes Etudes en Sciences Sociales in Paris. He is working on European kinship, paying particular attention to its cognatic character. The notion of the person inscribed in the kinship system and its implementations in the construction of social borders through the rhetoric of blood and genealogy have been at the centre of his publications. Now he is working on the continuities between the traditional kinship system and the situation generated by the new genetics. His publications include: 'Définitions des identités familiales chez les Xuetes de Majorque', in Patricia Hidiroglou (ed.) *Entre héritage et devenir. La construction de la famille juive* (Publications de la Sorbonne, 2003); 'Mujer, consensualismo y cognatismo, un sistema de parentesco en la historia', in Carmen Trillo San José (ed.), *Mujeres, familia y linaje en la Edad Media* (Ediciones de la Universidad de Granada, 2004).

Carles Salazar is Lecturer in Social Anthropology at the University of Lleida. He gained his PhD degree at the University of Cambridge, and has carried out ethnographic fieldwork in Ireland and Catalonia. His main research has been focused on different aspects of Irish society and culture: rural economy, religious beliefs, family organisation and history of sexual morality. He has also done research on the history of anthropology and on the cultural understanding of biomedicine and genetics among infertile couples. His latest publications include the book *Anthropology and Sexual Morality. A Theoretical Investigation* (Berghahn, 2006).

Jérôme Wilgaux teaches Greek history at the University of Nantes (France). He writes principally about kinship and marriage in ancient Greece. He was recently co-editor (with A. Bresson, M.P. Masson and S. Perentidis) of *Parenté et société dans le monde grec de l'Antiquité à l'âge moderne* (Bordeaux, 2006) and (with F. Prost) of *Penser et représenter le corps antique* (Presses universitaires de Rennes, 2006).

BIBLIOGRAPHY

Alber, E. 2003. 'Denying Biological Parenthood: Fosterage in Northern Benin', *Ethnos* 68 (4): 487–506.
Albee, E. 2004. *The Goat or 'Who Is Sylvia?'*. London: Methuen.
Allison, A. 1991. 'Japanese Mothers and "Obentos": the Lunch-box as Ideological State Apparatus', *Anthropological Quarterly* 64 (4): 195–208.
Anagnost, A. 2000. 'Scenes of Misrecognition: Maternal Citizenship in The Age of Transnational Adoption', *Positions-East Asia Cultures Critique* 8: 389–421.
APGL. 2001. *Aperçu sur les familles homoparentales. Enquête 2001 auprès des adhérents.* Association des Parents et Futurs Parents Gays et Lesbiens, htpp://www.apg.asso.fr
Aristotle. 1947. *Magna Moralia.* Loeb Classical Library no. 287. Cambridge MA: Harvard University Press.
────. 1979. *Generation of Animals*, trans. A.L. Peck. Cambridge: Harvard University Press.
Astuti, R. 2000. 'Kindreds and Descent Groups: New Perspectives from Madagascar', in J. Carsten (ed.), *Cultures of Relatedness: New Approaches to the Study of Kinship.* Cambridge: Cambridge University Press, pp. 90–103.
Bachelard, G. 1993. *La Formation de l'Esprit Scientifique* (1st edition 1938). Paris: Librairie Philosophique J. Vrin.
Barth, F. 2002. 'An Anthropology of Knowledge', *Current Anthropology* 43 (1): 1–18.
Bauer. M. and G. Gaskell (eds). 2002. *Biotechnology: the Making of a Global Controversy.* Cambridge: Cambridge University Press.
Bayne, T. and A. Kolers. 2003a. 'Parenthood and Procreation', in E.N. Zalta (ed.), *The Stanford Encyclopedia of Philosophy* (Spring 2003 edition). Retrieved 7 November 2005 from http://plato.stanford.edu/archives/spr2003/entries/parenthood/.
────. 2003b. 'Toward a Pluralist Account of Parenthood', *Bioethics* 17: 221–42.
Belmont, N. 1988. 'L'enfant et le fromage', *L'Homme* 105, XXVIII (1): 13–28.
Berdahl, D. 1999. *Where the World Ended: Re-unification and Identity in the German Borderland.* Berkeley: University of California Press.
Bestard, J. 1991. *What's in a Relative: Household and Family in Formentera.* New York and Oxford: Berg Publishers.
────. 1998. *Parentesco y Modernidad.* Barcelona: Paidós.
────. 2003. 'Naturaleza, cultura y parentesco: ¿naturalización de la cultura o genetificación de las relaciones?', in J.L. García and A. Barañano (eds), *Culturas en contacto. Encuentros y desencuentros.* Madrid: Ministerio de Educación, Cultura y Deporte, pp. 229–44.

———. 2004a. 'Kinship and the New Genetics. The Changing Meaning of Biogenetic Substance', *Social Anthropology* 12 (3): 253–63.

———. 2004b. *Tras la biología: La moralidad del parentesco y las nuevas tecnologías de reproducción*. Barcelona: Publicacions i Edicions de la Universitat de Barcelona.

Bestard, J., G. Orobitg, J. Ribot and C. Salazar. 2003. *Parentesco y Reproducción Asistida: Cuerpo, Persona y Relaciones*. Barcelona: Publicaciones de la Universitat de Barcelona.

Bock, J.D. 2000. 'Doing the Right Thing? Single Mothers by Choice and the Struggle for Legitimacy', *Gender and Society* 14 (1): 62–86.

Boholm, Å. 1983. *Swedish Kinship: an Exploration into Cultural Processes of Belonging and Continuity*. Göteborg Studies in Social Anthropology, 5. Göteborg: Acta Universitatis Gothoburgensis.

Boltanski, L. 2004. *La Condition fœtale. Une sociologie de l'engendrement et de l'avortement*. Paris: Gallimard.

Bomann-Larsen, T. 2004. *Haakon og Maud. Folket*, (Vol. 2). Oslo: Cappelen.

Bonnard, J.B. 2004. *Le Complexe de Zeus. Représentation de la paternité en Grèce ancienne*. Paris: Publications de la Sorbonne.

Borneman, J. 1992. *Belonging in the Two Berlins: Kin, State, Nation*. Cambridge: Cambridge University Press.

———. 2001. 'Caring and Being Cared for: Displacing Marriage, Kinship, Gender and Sexuality', in J.D. Faubion (ed.), *The Ethics of Kinship. Ethnographic Inquiries*. Lanban: Rowman and Littlefield, pp. 29–46.

Bouquet, M. 1993. *Reclaiming English Kinship: Portuguese Refractions of British Kinship Theory*. Manchester: Manchester University Press.

Bourdieu, P. 1977. *Outline of a Theory of Practice*. Cambridge: Cambridge University Press.

———. 2002. *Language and Symbolic Power*, 6th edn. Cambridge: Polity Press.

Cadoret, A. 1995. *Parenté plurielle. Anthropologie du placement familial*. Paris: L'Harmattan.

———. 2000. 'La parenté aujourd'hui: Agencement de la filiation et de l'alliance', *Sociétés contemporaines* 38: 5–19.

———. 2003. *Des parents comme les autres. Homosexualité et parenté*. Paris: Odile Jacob.

———. 2005. 'Une relecture de Schneider à la lumière des nouvelles familles', *Incidences* 1: 105–21.

Caplan, P. 1997. 'Approaches to the Study of Food, Health, and Identity', in P. Caplan (ed.), *Food, Health and Identity*. London: Routledge, pp. 1–31.

Carsten, J. 1995a. 'The Politics of Forgetting: Migration, Kinship and Memory on the Periphery of the Southeast Asian State', *Journal of the Royal Anthropological Institute* 1 (2): 317–35.

———. 1995b. 'The Substance of Kinship and the Heat of the Hearth: Feeding, Personhood, and Relatedness among Malays in Pulau Langkawi', *American Ethnologist* 22 (2): 223–41.

———. 1997. *The Heat of the Hearth: the Process of Kinship in a Malay Fishing Community*. Oxford: Clarendon Press.

———. (ed.). 2000a. *Cultures of Relatedness: New Approaches to the Study of Kinship*. Cambridge: Cambridge University Press.

———. 2000b. 'Knowing Where You've Come From: Ruptures and Continuities of Time and Kinship in Narratives of Adoption Reunions', *Journal of the Royal Anthropological Institute* 6: 687–703.

———. 2001. 'Substantivism, Antisubstantivism, and Anti-antisubstantivism', in S. Franklin and S. McKinnon (eds), *Relative Values. Reconfiguring Kinship Studies*, Durham and London: Duke University Press, pp. 29–53.

———. 2004. *After Kinship*. Cambridge: Cambridge University Press.

Cartwright, L. 2003. 'Photographs of "Waiting Children." The Transnational Adoption Market', *Social Text* 74 (21): 83–109.

Census of the Hungarian Central Statistical Office, 2001. Retrieved 7 November 2005 from http://www.nepszamlalas.hu/hun/kotetek/18/18_2_osszef.pdf.

Čepaitienė, A. 2003. 'Giminystė ir socialinis bei kultūrinis tapatumas dabartinėje Lietuvos visuomenėje (Kinship, and social and cultural identity in contemporary Lithuanian society)', *Lietuvių katalikų mokslo akademijos suvažiavimo darbai*, 18 (1): 197–207.

———. 2004. 'Conflicting memories: Personal life strategies and a vision of a state', in A. Paládi-Kovács (ed.), *Times, Places, Passages: Ethnological Approaches in the New Millennium*. Budapest: Akademiai Kiado, pp. 279–92.

Changeux, J.P. 2003. 'Introduction', in J.P. Changeux (ed.), *Gènes et Culture. Enveloppe génétique et variabilité culturelle*. Paris: Odile Jacob.

Clifford, J. 1986. 'Introduction: Partial Truths', in J. Clifford and G.E. Marcus (eds), *Writing Culture: the Poetics and Politics of Ethnography*. Berkeley, Los Angeles and London: University of California Press, pp. 1–26.

Coetzee, J.M. 1999. *The Lives of Animals*. Princeton: Princeton University Press.

Cohen, A. (ed.) 1982. *Belonging: Identity and Social Organisation in British Rural Cultures*. Manchester: Manchester University Press.

———. 1987. *Whalsay: Symbol, Segment and Boundary in a Shetland Island Community*. Manchester: Manchester University Press.

Conte, E. and C. Essner. 1995. *La Quête de la race. Une anthropologie du nazisme*. Paris: Hachette.

Coontz, S. 1992. *The Way We Never Were: American Families and the Nostalgia Trap*. New York: Basic Books

Counihan, C. 1999. *The Anthropology of Food and Body: Gender, Meaning and Power*. London: Routledge.

Courthiade, M. 2004. 'Kannauz on the Ganges, Cradle of the Romani People', in D. Kenrick (ed.), *Gypsies: from the Ganges to the Thames*. Hatfield, Hertfordshire: University of Hertfordshire Press, pp. 105–26.

Cousin, C. 1904. *De l'imprégnation de la mère (télégonie) d'après les données actuelles de la zootechnie*. Paris: H. Jouve.

Cussins, C. 1998. 'Producing Reproduction: Techniques of Normalization and Naturalization in Infertility Clinics', in S. Franklin and H. Ragoné (eds), *Reproducing Reproduction: Kinship, Power and Technological Innovation*. Philadelphia: University of Pennsylvania Press, pp. 66–101.

Dalton, S. 2000. 'Nonbiological Mothers and the Legal Boundaries of Motherhood. An Analysis of California Law', in H. Ragoné and F.W. Twine (eds), *Ideologies and Technologies of Motherhood. Race, Class, Sexuality, Nationalism*. London: Routledge, pp. 191–232.

Darr, A. 1997. 'Consanguineous Marriage and Genetics: a Positive Relationship', in A. Clarke and E. Parsons (eds), *Culture, Kinship and Genes. Towards Cross-cultural Genetics*. London: Macmillan, pp. 83–96.

Davison, C. 1997. 'Everyday Ideas of Inheritance and Health in Britain: Implications for Predictive Genetic Testing', in A. Clarke and E. Parsons (eds), *Culture, Kinship and Genes. Towards Cross-Cultural Genetics*. London: Macmillan, pp. 167–74.

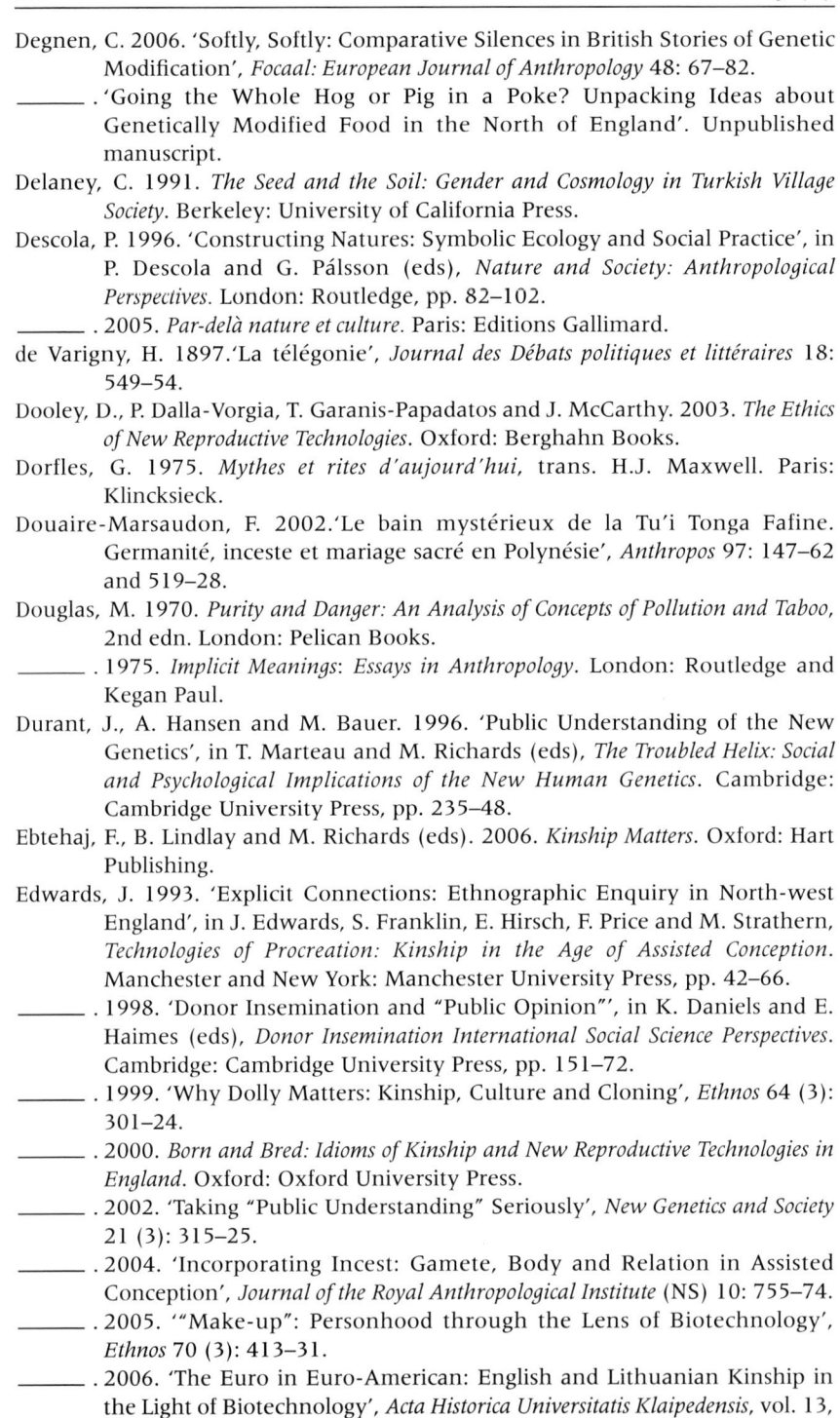

Degnen, C. 2006. 'Softly, Softly: Comparative Silences in British Stories of Genetic Modification', *Focaal: European Journal of Anthropology* 48: 67–82.

———. 'Going the Whole Hog or Pig in a Poke? Unpacking Ideas about Genetically Modified Food in the North of England'. Unpublished manuscript.

Delaney, C. 1991. *The Seed and the Soil: Gender and Cosmology in Turkish Village Society*. Berkeley: University of California Press.

Descola, P. 1996. 'Constructing Natures: Symbolic Ecology and Social Practice', in P. Descola and G. Pálsson (eds), *Nature and Society: Anthropological Perspectives*. London: Routledge, pp. 82–102.

———. 2005. *Par-delà nature et culture*. Paris: Editions Gallimard.

de Varigny, H. 1897.'La télégonie', *Journal des Débats politiques et littéraires* 18: 549–54.

Dooley, D., P. Dalla-Vorgia, T. Garanis-Papadatos and J. McCarthy. 2003. *The Ethics of New Reproductive Technologies*. Oxford: Berghahn Books.

Dorfles, G. 1975. *Mythes et rites d'aujourd'hui*, trans. H.J. Maxwell. Paris: Klincksieck.

Douaire-Marsaudon, F. 2002.'Le bain mystérieux de la Tu'i Tonga Fafine. Germanité, inceste et mariage sacré en Polynésie', *Anthropos* 97: 147–62 and 519–28.

Douglas, M. 1970. *Purity and Danger: An Analysis of Concepts of Pollution and Taboo*, 2nd edn. London: Pelican Books.

———. 1975. *Implicit Meanings: Essays in Anthropology*. London: Routledge and Kegan Paul.

Durant, J., A. Hansen and M. Bauer. 1996. 'Public Understanding of the New Genetics', in T. Marteau and M. Richards (eds), *The Troubled Helix: Social and Psychological Implications of the New Human Genetics*. Cambridge: Cambridge University Press, pp. 235–48.

Ebtehaj, F., B. Lindlay and M. Richards (eds). 2006. *Kinship Matters*. Oxford: Hart Publishing.

Edwards, J. 1993. 'Explicit Connections: Ethnographic Enquiry in North-west England', in J. Edwards, S. Franklin, E. Hirsch, F. Price and M. Strathern, *Technologies of Procreation: Kinship in the Age of Assisted Conception*. Manchester and New York: Manchester University Press, pp. 42–66.

———. 1998. 'Donor Insemination and "Public Opinion"', in K. Daniels and E. Haimes (eds), *Donor Insemination International Social Science Perspectives*. Cambridge: Cambridge University Press, pp. 151–72.

———. 1999. 'Why Dolly Matters: Kinship, Culture and Cloning', *Ethnos* 64 (3): 301–24.

———. 2000. *Born and Bred: Idioms of Kinship and New Reproductive Technologies in England*. Oxford: Oxford University Press.

———. 2002. 'Taking "Public Understanding" Seriously', *New Genetics and Society* 21 (3): 315–25.

———. 2004. 'Incorporating Incest: Gamete, Body and Relation in Assisted Conception', *Journal of the Royal Anthropological Institute* (NS) 10: 755–74.

———. 2005. '"Make-up": Personhood through the Lens of Biotechnology', *Ethnos* 70 (3): 413–31.

———. 2006. 'The Euro in Euro-American: English and Lithuanian Kinship in the Light of Biotechnology', *Acta Historica Universitatis Klaipedensis*, vol. 13, *Studia Antropologica 2*, Klaipeda: Klaipeda University Publisher, pp. 129–39.

_____. 2008. *The Social Life of Blood and Genes*. Paris: École des Hautes Études en Sciences Sociales (EHESS).

_____. n.d. 'PUG in PUS'. Unpublished manuscript.

Edwards, J. and M. Strathern. 2000. 'Including our Own', in J. Carsten (ed.), *Cultures of Relatedness: New Approaches to the Study of Kinship*. Cambridge: Cambridge University Press, pp. 149–66.

Edwards, J., S. Franklin, E. Hirsch, F. Price and M. Strathern.1993. *Technologies of Procreation: Kinship in the Age of Assisted Conception*. Manchester and New York: Manchester University Press.

Edwards, J., P. Harvey and P. Wade (eds) 2007. *Anthropology and Science: Epistemologies in Practice*. Oxford: Berg.

Edwards, J., P. Harvey and P. Wade (eds) 2008. *Technologized Images, Technologized Bodies: Anthropological Approaches to a New Politics of Vision*. Oxford and New York: Berghahn Books.

Elster, J. 1977. 'Ulysses and the Sirens: a Theory of Imperfect Rationality', *Social Science Information* XVI (5): 469–526.

ESRC. 1999. *The Politics of GM Foods*. Swindon: ESRC.

Evans, J.H. 2002. *Playing God? Human Genetics Engineering and the Rationalization of Public Bioethical Debate*. Chicago: University of Chicago Press.

Evans-Pritchard, E.E. 1940. *The Nuer. A Description of the Modes of Livelihood and Political Institutions of a Nilotic People*. Oxford and New York: Oxford University Press.

Faubion, J. (ed.). 2001. *The Ethics of Kinship: Ethnographic Inquiries*. Lanham, MD: Rowman and Littlefield.

Featherstone, K., P. Atkinson, P. Bharadwaj and A. Clarke. 2006. *Risky Relations: Family, Kinship and the New Genetics*. Oxford: Berg.

Feeley-Harnik, G. 2001. 'The Ethnography of Creation: Lewis Henry Morgan and the American Beaver', in S. Franklin and S. McKinnon (eds), *Relative Values: Reconfiguring Kinship Studies*. Durham: Duke University Press, pp. 54–84.

_____. 2004. 'The Geography of Descent', *Proceedings of the British Academy*, vol. 125. Oxford: Oxford University Press, pp. 312–64.

Feinberg, R. and M. Ottenheimer (eds). 2001. *The Cultural Analysis of Kinship. The Legacy of David M. Schneider*. Urbana and Chicago: University of Illinois Press.

Fineman, M.A. 1995. *The Neutered Mother, the Sexual Family and Other Twentieth Century Tragedies*. New York: Routledge.

Finkler, K. 2000. *Experiencing the New Genetics. Family and Kinship on the Medical Frontier*. Philadelphia: University of Pennsylvania Press.

_____. 2001. 'The Kin in the Gene. The Medicalization of Family and Kinship in American Society', *Current Anthropology* 42: 235–63.

Flandrin, J.L. 1981. 'Les créantailles troyennes (XVe – XVIIe siècle)', in J.L. Flandrin (ed.), *Le Sexe et l'Occident. Evolution des attitudes et des comportements*. Paris: Seuil, pp. 61–82.

Fortier, C. 2001. 'Le lait, le sperme, le dos. Et le sang? Représentations physiologiques de la filiation et de la parenté de lait en Islam malékite et dans la société maure de Mauritanie', *Cahiers d'Études Africaines* 161 (XL-1): 97–138.

Foucault, M. 1981. *The History of Sexuality*. Vol. 1. Harmondsworth: Penguin.

_____. 1991. 'Governmentality', in G. Burchell, C. Gordon and P. Miller (eds), *The Foucault Effect: Studies in Governmentality*. Chicago: University of Chicago Press, pp. 87–104.

_____. 1998. *A fantasztikus könyvtár*. Budapest: Pallas Stúdió/Attraktor KFT.

_____. 2003. *Le Pouvoir psychiatrique. Cours au Collège de France, 1973–74*. Paris: Hautes Études, Gallimard, Seuil.

Fourmont, M. 2003. 'Couple frère et sœur', documentary for the programme *Incroyable mais vrai*. TF1, R&G Productions.

Franklin, S. 1993. 'Making Representations: the Parliamentary Debate on the Human Fertilisation and Embryology Act', in J. Edwards, S. Franklin, E. Hirsch, F. Price and M. Strathern (eds), *Technologies of Procreation. Kinship in the Age of Assisted Conception*. Manchester: Manchester University Press, pp. 96–131.

_____. 1997. *Embodied Progress: a Cultural Account of Assisted Conception*. London: Routledge.

_____. 2001. 'Biologization Revisited: Kinship Theory in the Context of the New Biologies', in S. Franklin and S. McKinnon (eds), *Relative Values: Reconfiguring Kinship Studies*. Durham: Duke University Press, pp. 302–25.

_____. 2003. 'Re-thinking Nature-Culture: Anthropology and the New Genetics', *Anthropological Theory* 3 (1): 65–85.

Franklin, S. and S. McKinnon. 2001. 'Introduction', in S. Franklin and S. McKinnon, (eds), *Relative Values. Reconfiguring Kinship Studies*. Durham: Duke University Press, pp. 1–25.

Freud, S. 2003 [1920] *La psicología de las masas*. Madrid: Alianza.

Fukuyama, F. 2002. *Our Posthuman Future: Consequences of the Biotechnology Revolution*. London: Profile.

Gamella, J. 1996. *La población gitana en Andalucía*. Sevilla: Junta de Andalucía.

García Marín, J.M. 1980. *El aborto criminal en la legislación y la doctrina (pasado y presente de una polémica)*. Madrid: Editoriales de derecho reunidas.

Gay y Blasco, P. 1999. *Gypsies in Madrid. Sex, Gender and the Performance of Identity*. Oxford and New York: Berg.

Geertz, C. 1983. *Local Knowledge: Further Essays in Interpretive Anthropology*. London: Fontana Press.

Gellner, E. 1973. *The Concept of Kinship*. Oxford: Blackwell.

Ginsburg, F.D. and R. Rapp (eds). 1995. *Conceiving the New World Order: The Global Politics of Reproduction*. Berkeley: University of California Press.

Gmeiner, H. 1993. *Az SOS Gyermekfalavak*. Innsbruck-Munich: SOS Kinderdorf Press.

Godelier, M. 1982. *La Production des grands hommes*. Paris: Fayard.

_____. 2004. *Métamorphoses de la parenté*. Paris: Fayard.

Goodenough, W.H. 2001. 'Muddles in Schneider's Model', in R. Feinberg and M. Ottenheimer (eds), *The Cultural Analysis of Kinship. The Legacy of David M. Schneider*. Urbana and Chicago: University of Chicago Press, pp. 205–18.

Goody, J. 1976. *Production and Reproduction: a Comparative Study of the Domestic Domain*. Cambridge: Cambridge University Press.

Green, S. 2002. 'Culture in a Network: Dykes, Webs and Women in London and Manchester', in N. Rapport (ed.), *British Subjects: an Anthropology of Britain*. Oxford: Berg, pp. 181–202.

Grove-White, R., P. Macnaghten, S. Mayer and B. Wynne. 1997. *Uncertain World: Genetically Modified Organisms, Food and Public Attitudes in Britain*. Lancaster: CSEC.

Grove-White, R., P. Macnaghten and B. Wynne. 2000. *Wising Up: the Public and New Technologies*. Lancaster: CSEC.

Gudeman, S. 1976. *Relationships, Residence and the Individual: a Rural Panamanian Community*. London: Routledge and Kegan Paul.

Gullestad, M. 1984. *Kitchen-table Society. A Case Study of the Family Life and Friendships of Young Working-class Mothers in Urban Norway*. Oslo: Universitetsforlaget.

Gullestad, M. and M. Segalen. 1995. *La Famille en Europe. Parenté et perpétuation familiale*. Paris: La Découverte.

Haimes, E. 1992. 'Gamete Donation and the Social Management of Genetic Origins', in M. Stacey (ed.), *Changing Human Reproduction. Social Science Perspectives*. Sage Publications: London, pp. 119–47.

Haraway, D. 1991. *Simians, Cyborgs and Women: the Reinvention of Nature*. New York: Routledge.

―――. 1997. *Modest_Witness@Second_Millenium.FemaleMan©_meets oncomouse [tm]: Feminism and Technoscience*. New York: Routledge.

Harris, C.C. 1990. *Kinship*. Minneapolis: University of Minnesota Press.

Hastrup, K. 1996. 'Anthropological Theory as Practice', *Social Anthropology* 4 (1): 75–81.

Hastrup, K. and P. Hervik. 1994. 'Introduction', in K. Hastrup and P. Hervik (eds), *Social Experience and Anthropological Knowledge*. London: Routledge, pp. 1–12.

Hayden, C. 1995. 'Gender, Genetics and Generation: Reformulating Biology in Lesbian Kinship', *Cultural Anthropology* 10 (1): 41–64.

Heller, C. 2002. 'From Scientific Risk to *Paysan* Savoir-faire: Peasant Expertise in the French and Global Debate over GM Crops', *Science as Culture* 11 (1): 5–37.

Helmreich, S. 2001. 'Kinship in Hypertext: Transubstantiating Fatherhood and Information Flow in Artificial Life', in S. Franklin and S. McKinnon (eds), *Relative Values: Reconfiguring Kinship Studies*. Durham: Duke University Press, pp. 116–43.

Héritier, F. 1977. 'L'identité Samo', in *L'Identité. Séminaire interdisciplinaire dirigé par C. Lévi-Strauss*. Paris: Quadrige/PUF, pp. 51–80.

―――. 1981. *L'Exercice de la parenté*. Paris: Hautes Etudes/Gallimard/Le Seuil.

―――. 1994. *Les Deux Sœurs et leur mère*. Paris: Odile Jacob.

―――. 1996. *Masculin/Féminin. La Pensée de la différence*. Paris: Odile Jacob.

Hermida, X. and X.M. Pereiro. 1997. 'Una pareja de hermanos con hijos abrirá el registro de uniones de hecho de Cambre', *El País*, 3 April.

Hertz, R. 2002. 'The Father as an Idea: a Challenge to Kinship Boundaries by Single Mothers', *Symbolic Interaction* 25 (1): 1–31.

Hill, J.H. and B. Mannheim.1992. 'Language and Worldview', *Annual Review of Anthropology* 21: 381–406.

Hirsch, E. 1993. 'Negotiated Limits: Interviews in South-East England', in J. Edwards, S. Franklin, E. Hirsch, F. Price and M. Strathern, *Technologies of Procreation: Kinship in the Age of Assisted Conception*. Manchester and New York: Manchester University Press, pp. 67–95.

Hocart, A.M. 1968 [1937]. 'Kinship Systems', in P. Bohannan and J. Middleton (eds), *Kinship and Social Organization*. New York: Natural History Press, pp. 29–38.

Hoffman-Reim, C. 1990. *The Adopted Child: Family Life with Double Parenthood*. London: Transaction Publishers.

Holy, L. 1996. *Anthropological Perspectives on Kinship*. London and Chicago: Pluto Press.
Howell, S. 2001. 'Self-conscious Kinship: Some Contested Values in Norwegian Transnational Adoption', in S. Franklin and S. McKinnon (eds), *Relative Values. Reconfiguring Kinship Studies*. Durham: Duke University Press, pp. 203–23.
———. 2003. 'Kinning: The Creation of Life-trajectories in Adoptive Families', *Journal of the Royal Anthropological Institute* (NS) 9 (3): 465–84.
———. 2006. The Kinning of Foreigners: Transnational Adoption in a Global Perspective. Oxford and New York: Berghahn Books.
Howell, S. and D. Marre. 2006. 'To Kin a Transnationally Adopted Child in Norway and Spain: the Achievement of Resemblances and Belonging', *Ethnos* 71 (3): 293–316.
Howell, S. and M. Melhuus. 1993. 'The Study of Kinship; the Study of Person; a Study of Gender?', in T. del Valle (ed.), *Gendered Anthropology*. London and New York: Routledge, pp. 38–53.
Howell, S. and M. Melhuus (eds). 2001. *Blod – tykkere enn vann? Betydninger av slektskap i Norge*. Bergen: Fagbokforlaget.
Howell, S. and M. Melhuus. 2007. 'Mixed Race Families – Do They Exist? Some Criteria for Identity and Belonging in Contemporary Norway', in P. Wade (ed.), *Race, Ethnicity and Nation: Perspectives from Kinship and Genetics*. Oxford: Berghahn.
http://www.angelcovers.org/ccaaset2.shtml.
http://www.comlaw.gov.au/ComLaw/Legislation/LegislativeInstrument Compilation1.
http://www.dagbladet.no/?/nyheter/2004/10/14/411285.html.
http://www.familyoffour.homestead.com/June05CCAA.html.
Hungarian Act No. XXXI of 1997 on Child Protection.
Iacub, M. 2004. *L'Empire du ventre. Pour une autre histoire de la maternité*. Paris: Fayard.
Ingold, T. 1996. 'Hunting and Gathering as Ways of Perceiving the Environment', in R. Ellen and K. Fukui (eds), *Redefining Nature: Ecology, Culture and Domestication*. Oxford: Berg, pp. 117–55.
Ingvaldsen, S. 1996. *Rette foreldre og virkelige barn: Norsk adopsjonslovgivning 1917 – 1986*. Universitet i Bergen, Bergen: hovedfagsoppgave i historie.
Jacob, F. 1972. *La Logique du vivant*. Paris: Gallimard.
Jasanoff, S. (ed.). 2004. *States of Knowledge: the Co-production of Science and Social Order*. London and New York: Routledge.
Jeddi, A. 2003. 'Falling Between Two Stools. The Relationship Between SOS Children's Village Families and the Biological Families', *SOS Kinderdorforum* 27: 8–11.
Jeudy-Ballini, M. 1992. 'De la filiation en plus: l'adoption chez les Sulka de Nouvelle Bretagne', *Droit et cultures* 23: 109–35.
Jones, B.D. 2003. 'Single Motherhood by Choice, Libertarian Feminism and the Uniform Parentage Act', *Texas Journal of Women and the Law* 12: 419–49.
Jones, S. 2000. *Almost Like a Whale: the Origin of Species Updated*. London: Anchor.
Kahn, S.M. 2000. *Reproducing Jews. A Cultural Account of Assisted Conception in Israel*. Durham: Duke University Press.
———. 2002. 'The Uses of New Reproductive Technologies among Ultraorthodox Jews in Israel', in M.C. Inhorn and F. van Balen (eds), *Infertility Around the Globe. New Thinking on Childlessness, Gender and Reproductive Technologies*. Berkeley: University of California Press, pp. 283–97.

Kapitány, B. 2003. 'Az értékbeállítódások különbségei különböző kohorszokban és életkorokban', in Zs. Spéder (ed.), *Család és népesség – itthon és Európában*. Budapest: Századvég Kiadó – KSH Népességtudományi Kutatóintézet, pp. 254–78.

Knorr-Cetina, K. 1999. *Epistemic Cultures: How the Sciences Make Knowledge*. Cambridge Mass.: Harvard University Press.

Konrad, M. 1998. 'Ova Donation and Symbols of Substance: Some Variations on the Theme of Sex, Gender and the Partible Body', *Journal of the Royal Anthropological Institute* (NS) 4: 643–67.

———. 2003. 'From Secrets of Life to the Life of Secrets: Tracing Genetic Knowledge as Genealogical Ethics in Biomedical Britain', *Journal of the Royal Anthropological Institute* (NS) 9: 339–58.

———. 2005. *Nameless Relations. Anonymity, Melanesia and Reproductive Gift Exchange between British Ova Donors and Recipients*. New York and Oxford: Berghahn Books.

Krusiewicz, E.S. and J.T. Wood. 2001. '"He Was Our Child from the Moment We Walked In that Room": Entrance Stories of Adoptive Parents', *Journal of Social and Personal Relationships* 18: 785–803.

Kuper, A. 1999. *Culture: the Anthropologists' Account*. Cambridge, Mass.: Harvard University Press.

———. 2002. 'Incest, Cousin Marriage and the Origin of the Human Sciences in Nineteenth-century England', *Past and Present* 174: 158–83.

Labby, D. 1976. 'Incest as Cannibalism: the Yapese Analysis', *Journal of the Polynesian Society* 85 (2): 171–80.

Lagunas Arias, D. 2000. 'Dentro de "Dentro": Estudio Antropológico y Social de una Comunidad de Gitanos Catalanes', PhD dissertation, University of Jaén.

Laqueur, T. 1990. *Making Sex: Body and Gender from the Greeks to Freud*. Cambridge: Harvard University Press.

Latour, B. 1991. *Nous n'avons pas été modernes*. Paris: La Decouverte.

———. 2004. *The Politics of Nature: How to Bring the Sciences into Democracy*. Cambridge: Harvard University Press.

———. 2005. *Reassembling the Social*. Oxford: Oxford University Press.

Leach, E. 1961. *Pul Eliya, a Village in Ceylon: a Study of Land Tenure and Kinship*. Cambridge: Cambridge University Press.

———. 1969. 'Virgin Birth', in E.R. Leach, *Genesis as Myth and Other Essays*. London: Jonathan Cape, pp. 85–119.

Leaf, M.J. 2001. 'Schneider's Idealism, Relativism, and the Confusion of Kinship', in R. Feinberg and M. Ottenheimer (eds), *The Cultural Analysis of Kinship. The Legacy of David M. Schneider*. Urbana and Chicago: University of Chicago Press, pp. 60–77.

Legrand, C. 2004. 'Le Négoce de la parenté. De la quête de parenté dans l'Irlande contemporaine', PhD dissertation, École des Hautes Études en Sciences Sociales (EHESS), Paris.

Leira, A. 1996. *Parents, Children and the State: Family Obligations in Norway*. Oslo: Institute for Social Research.

Leitch, A. 2003. 'Slow Food and the Politics of Pork Fat: Italian Food and European Identity', *Ethnos* 68 (4): 437–62.

Le Roy Ladurie, E. 1980. *Montaillou*. Harmondsworth: Penguin Books.

Lévai, K. 2000. *A nő szerint a világ*. Budapest: Osiris Zsebkönyvtár.

Levidow, L. 2002. 'Ignorance-based Risk Assessment? Scientific Controversy over GM Food Safety', *Science as Culture* 11 (1): 61–67.

Lévi-Strauss, C. 1962. *La Pensée sauvage*. Paris: Plon.
———. 1969. *The Elementary Structures of Kinship*, trans. J.H. Bell and J.R. von Sturmer. Boston: Beacon Press.
———. 1973 [1962]. *Totemism*. Harmondsworth: Penguin.
———. 1977. *Structural Anthropology*, Vol. II, trans. M. Layton. London: Penguin Books.
Lévi-Strauss, C. and D. Éribon. 1988. *De près et de loin*. Paris: Odile Jacob.
Lewin, E. 1993. *Lesbian Mothers*. Ithaca, New York: Cornell University Press.
Lezaun, J. 2004. 'Subjects of Knowledge: Epistemologies of the Consumer in the GM Food Debate', in N. Stehr (ed.), *The Governance of Knowledge*. London: Transaction Publishers, pp. 187–206.
Lietuvių kalbos žodynas (Dictionary of Lithuanian Language).1956. Vol. 3, Vilnius: Valstybinė politinės ir mokslinės literatūros leidykla; 1981. Vol. 12, Vilnius: Mokslas; 1986. Vol. 14, Vilnius: Mokslas.
Lippman, A. 1992. 'Mother Matters: a Fresh look at Prenatal Genetic Testing', *Journal in Reproductive and Genetic Medicine*, 5 (2): 141–54.
Løvset, J. 1951. 'Artificial Insemination. The Attitude of Patients in Norway', *Fertility and Sterility* 2 (5): 414–29.
MacCormack, C. and M. Strathern (eds). 1980. *Nature, Culture and Gender*. Cambridge: Cambridge University Press.
Malinowski, B. 1932. *The Sexual Life of Savages in North-western Melanesia*. London: Routledge and Kegan Paul.
Manrique, N. 2004. 'La lune pétrifiée. Représentations parthénogénétiques dans une communauté gitane (Grenade)', in F. Héritier and M. Xanthakou (eds), *Corps et Affects*. Paris: Odile Jacob, pp. 205–20.
Martin, E. 1991. 'The Egg and the Sperm: How Science Has Constructed a Romance Based on Stereotypical Male-Female Roles', *Signs: Journal of Women in Culture and Society* 16 (3): 485–501.
———. 1994. *Flexible Bodies: the Role of Immunity in American Culture from the Days of Polio to the Age of AIDS*. Boston: Beacon Press.
Martínez, A. 2004. 'El largo y costoso proceso de la adopción', *Expansión* 23 February. Madrid.
Mathieu, N.C. 1991. *L'Anatomie politique. Catégorisations et idéologies du sexe*. Paris: Côté-femmes.
McKinley, R. 2001. 'The Philosophy of Kinship: a Reply to Schneider's Critique of the Study of Kinship', in R. Feinberg and M. Ottenheimer (eds), *The Cultural Analysis of Kinship. The Legacy of David M. Schneider*. Urbana and Chicago: University of Chicago Press, pp. 131–67.
McKinnon, S. and S. Silverman (eds). 2005. *Complexities: Beyond Nature and Nurture*. Chicago: University of Chicago Press.
Meillassoux, C. 2000. 'Construire et déconstruire la parenté', *Sociétés Contemporaines* 38: 37–47.
Melhuus, M. 2001. 'Kan skinnet bedra? Noen meninger om assistert befruktning i Norge', in S. Howell and M. Melhuus (eds), *Blod – tykkere enn vann? Betydninger av slektskap i Norge*. Bergen: Fagbokforlaget.
———. 2003. 'Exchange Matters. Issues of Law and the Flow of Human Substances', in T.H. Eriksen (ed.), *Globalisation. Studies in Anthropology*. London: Pluto Press, pp. 170–97.
———. 2005a. '"Better Safe Than Sorry". Legislating Assisted Conception in Norway', in C. Krohn-Hansen and K. Nustad (eds), *State Formation. Anthropological Perspectives*. London: Pluto, pp. 212–33.

———. 2005b. 'Biotechnology and Fundamental Notions of Relatedness and Society. An Exploration of the Norwegian Notion of "Sorting Society"'. Paper presented at the conference, Vital Matters. Biotechnology and its Social and Ethical Implications. Bergen.

———. Forthcoming. 'Procreative Imaginations. When Experts Disagree on the Meanings of Kinship', in M.E. Lien and M. Melhuus (eds), *Holding Worlds Together. Ethnographies of Knowing and Belonging*. Oxford: Berghahn Books.

Messer, E. 1984. 'Anthropological Perspectives on Diet', *Annual Review of Anthropology* 13: 205–49.

Ministry of Justice. 1953. *Instilling fra inseminasjonskomitéen*. Oslo.

Mintz, S. and C. Du Bois. 2002. 'The Anthropology of Food and Eating', *Annual Review of Anthropology* 31: 99–119.

Miró, A. 2003. *La hija del Ganges. Historia de una adopción*. Barcelona: Lumen.

———. 2004. *Las dos caras de la luna*. Barcelona: Lumen.

Modell, J. 1994. *Kinship with Strangers: Adoption and Interpretations of Kinship in American Culture*. Berkeley: University of California Press.

———. 2002. *A Sealed and Secret Kinship: the Culture of Policies and Practices in American Adoption*. Oxford: Berghahn Books.

Moore, H. 1994. *A Passion for Difference. Essays in Anthropology and Gender*. Cambridge: Polity Press.

Moscovici, S. 1995. 'Fenomenul reprezentărilor sociale', in A. Neculau (ed.), *Reprezentările sociale*. Bucharest: Știință & Tehnică, pp. 1–84.

Murcott, A. 1999. '"Not Science but PR": GM Food and the Makings of a Considered Sociology', *Sociological Research Online* 4 (3).

Myerson, G. 2000. *Donna Haraway and GM Foods*. Cambridge: Icon Books.

Nash, C. 2002. 'Genealogical Identities', *Environment and Planning* 20: 27–52.

Needham, R. 1971. 'Remarks on the Analysis of Kinship and Marriage', in R. Needham (ed.), *Rethinking Kinship and Marriage*. London: Tavistock Publications, pp. 1–34.

Nelkin, D. and M.S. Lindee. 1995. *The DNA Mystique. The Gene as a Cultural Icon*. New York: W.H. Freeman.

Neményi, M. 1995. 'The Social Representation of Step Families', in U. Bjornberg (ed.), *European Parents in the 1990s*. New Brunswick: Transaction Publishers, pp. 243–56.

———. 2000. *Csoportkép nőkkel*. Budapest: Új Mandátum Könyvkiadó.

Nowotny, H., P. Scott and M. Gibbon. 2001. *Rethinking Science. Knowledge and the Public in an Age of Uncertainty*. Cambridge: Polity Press.

Okely, J. 1983. *The Travellers-Gypsies*. Cambridge: Cambridge University Press.

Orobitg, G. and C. Salazar. 2005. 'The Gift of Motherhood: Egg Donation in a Barcelona Infertility Clinic', *Ethnos* 70 (1): 31–52.

Ortiz, A.M. 2005. 'Incesto/Del mito a la vida. Hermanos, pareja y padres', *El Mundo*, supplement 495, 10 April.

Ottenheimer, M. 2001. 'Relativism in Kinship Analysis', in R. Feinberg and M. Ottenheimer (eds) *The Cultural Analysis of Kinship. The Legacy of David M. Schneider*. Urbana and Chicago: University of Illinois Press, pp. 118–30.

Oudshoorn, N. 1994. *Beyond the Natural Body: an Archaeology of Sex Hormones*. London: Routledge.

Pálsson, G. and K.E. Hardardóttir. 2002 'From Whom the Cell Tolls. Debates about Biomedicine', *Current Anthropology* 43: 271–301.

Parkin, R. and L. Stone (eds). 2004. *Kinship and Family: an Anthropological Reader*. Oxford: Blackwell.

Pasqualino, C. 1998. *Dire le chant. Les Gitans flamencos d'Andalousie.* Paris: CNRS Éditions and Éditions de la Maison des Sciences de L'Homme.
Paukštytė, R. 1999. *Gimtuvės ir krikštynos Lietuvos kaimo gyvenime (XIX a. pabaigoje – XX a. pirmoje pusėje) (Childbirth and Baptism in Lithuanian Village Life at the end of the 19th and the first half of the 20th century).* Vilnius: Diemedžio leidykla.
Peirce, C.S. 1965. *Collected Papers.* Cambridge, Mass.: Harvard University Press.
Peletz, M.G. 1995. 'Kinship Studies in Late Twentieth-century Anthropology', *Annual Review of Anthropology* 24: 343–72.
Pina-Cabral, J. 2002. *O homem na família. Cinco ensaios de antropología.* Lisbon: Imprensa de Ciências Sociais.
Plato. 1991. *The Republic: the Complete and Unabridged Jowett Translation.* New York: Vintage Classic Edition.
Pliny. 1969. *Natural History in Ten Volumes.* Vol. II. Cambridge, Mass.: Harvard University Press.
Pocius, G.L. 1991. *A Place to Belong: Community Order and Everyday Space in Calvert, Newfoundland.* Athens and London: University of Georgia Press, Montreal and Kingston: McGill-Queen's University Press.
Pollan, M. 2001. *The Botany of Desire: a Plant's-eye View of the World.* New York: Random House.
Poly, J.-P. 2003. *Le Chemin des amours barbares. Genèse médiévale de la sexualité européenne.* Paris: Perrin.
Pongrácz, T. and E. Molnár. 1997. 'A gyermekvállalási magatartás alakulása', in K. Lévai and I.Gy. Tóth (eds), *Szerepváltozások. Jelentés a nők helyzetéről.* Budapest: Tárki, pp. 86–103.
Porqueres i Gené, E. 2000. 'Cognatisme et voies du sang. La créativité du mariage canonique', *L'Homme* 154–55: 335–56.
——. 2004. 'Individu et parenté. Individuation de l'embryon', in F. Héritier and M. Xanthakou (eds), *Corps et Affects.* Paris: Odile Jacob, pp. 139–50.
Poutignat, P. and J. Streiff-Fenart. 1995. *Théories de l'ethnicité.* Paris: Presses Universitaires de France.
Rabinow, P. 1992. 'Artificiality and Enlightenment: From Sociobiology to Biosociality', in J. Crary and S. Kwinter (eds), *Incorporations.* New York: Zone Books, pp. 234–52.
——. 1996. *Essays on the Anthropology of Reason.* Princeton, NJ: Princeton University Press.
Ragoné, H. 1994. *Surrogate Motherhood. Conception in the Heart.* Boulder: Westview Press.
——. 1999. 'The Gift of Life. Surrogate Motherhood, Gamete Donation, and Construction of Altruism', in *Transformative Motherhood. On Giving and Getting in a Consumer Culture.* New York and London: New York University Press, pp. 65–88.
——. 2000. 'Of Likeness and Difference: How Race is Being Transfigured by Gestational Surrogacy', in H. Ragoné and F. Winddance Twine (eds), *Ideologies and Technologies of Motherhood: Race, Class, Sexuality and Nationalism.* New York and London: Routledge, pp. 56–75.
Rapp, R. 1999. *Testing the Women. Testing the Foetus.* London: Routledge.
Rapp, R., D. Heath and K.S. Taussig. 2001. 'Genealogical Dis-Ease: Where Hereditary Abnormality, Biomedical Explanation, and Family Responsibility Meet', in S. Franklin and S. McKinnon (eds), *Relative Values. Reconfiguring Kinship Studies.* Durham: Duke University Press, pp. 384–409.

Rappaport, R.A. 1968. *Pigs for the Ancestors. Ritual in the Ecology of a New Guinea People*. New Haven and London: Yale University Press.
Rausing, S. 2004. *History, Memory and Identity in Post-Soviet Estonia*. Oxford: Oxford University Press.
Read, D.W. 2001. 'What is Kinship', in R. Feinberg and M. Ottenheimer (eds), *The Cultural Analysis of Kinship. The Legacy of David M. Schneider*. Urbana and Chicago: University of Chicago Press, pp. 78–117.
Reilly, J. and D. Miller. 1997. 'Scaremonger or Scapegoat? The Role of the Media in the Emergence of Food as a Social Issue', in P. Caplan (ed.), *Food, Health and Identity*. London: Routledge, pp. 234–51.
Reynolds, H.B. 1978. '"To Keep the Tali Strong": Women's Rituals in Tamilnad, India', PhD dissertation, University of Wisconsin.
Rheinberger, H.J. 2000. 'Beyond Nature and Culture: Modes of Reasoning in the Age of Molecular Biology and Medicine', in M. Lock, A. Young and A. Cambrosio (eds), *Living and Working with the New Medical Technologies. Intersection of Inquiry*. Cambridge: Cambridge University Press, pp. 19–30.
Richards, M. 1997. 'It Runs in the Family: Lay Knowledge about Inheritance', in A. Clarke and E. Parsons (eds), *Culture, Kinship and Genes. Towards Cross-cultural Genetics*. London: Macmillan, pp. 175–94.
Ricoeur, P. 1992. *Oneself as Another*, trans. K. Blamey. Chicago: Chicago University Press.
——— . 2000. *Interpretacijos teorija: diskursas ir reikšmės perteklius (Interpretation Theory: Discourse and the Surplus of Meaning)*, trans. R. Kalinauskaitė and G. Lidžiuvienė. Vilnius: Baltos lankos.
Roll-Hansen, N. and G. Broberg (eds). 1996. *Eugenics and the Welfare State: Sterilization Policy in Denmark, Sweden, Norway and Finland*. East Lancing: Michigan University Press.
Rønne-Pettersen, E. 1951. *Prövrörsmänniskan. En studie i moderne magi*. Stockholm: Bokförlaget biopsykologi.
Roscoe, P.B. 1994. 'Amity and Aggression: a Symbolic Theory of Incest', *Man* (NS) 29 (1): 49–76.
Rose, N. 1999. *Governing the Soul: The Shaping of the Private Self*. London: Free Association Books.
Rose, S. 1998. *Lifelines: Biology, Freedom, Determinism*. London: Penguin Books.
Rubin, G. 1975. 'The Traffic In Women: Notes on the "Political Economy" of Sex', in R.R. Reiter (ed.) *Toward an Anthropology of Women*. New York: Monthly Review Press, pp. 157–210.
Salazar, C. 1999. 'On Blood and its Alternatives. An Irish History', *Social Anthropology* 7 (2): 155 67.
——— . 2004. 'Primordial Obligations: an Exploration of the Moral Basis of Western Kinship Systems', *Journal of the Society for the Anthropology of Europe* 4 (1): 16–23.
——— . 2006. *Anthropology and Sexual Morality. A Theoretical Investigation*. Oxford and New York: Berghahn Books.
Sandemose, A. 1952. 'Unnfanget i løgn', *Årstidene* 2: 24–86.
Scheffler, H.W. 1991. 'Sexism and Naturalism in the Study of Kinship', in M. Di Leonardo (ed.), *Gender at the Crossroads of Knowledge: Feminist Anthropology in the Postmodern Era*. Berkeley: University of California Press, pp. 361–82.
Schlee, G. 2004. 'Taking Sides and Constructing Identities: Reflections on Conflict Theory', *Journal of Royal Anthropological Institute* 10: 135–56.

Schneider, D.M. 1957. 'Political Organization, Supernatural Sanctions and the Punishment for Incest on Yap', *American Anthropologist* 59: 791–800.
——— . 1968. *American Kinship: a Cultural Account*. Chicago: University of Chicago Press.
——— . 1976. 'The Meaning of Incest', *Journal of the Polynesian Society* 85 (2): 149–69.
——— . 1984. *A Critique of the Study of Kinship*. Ann Arbor: University of Michigan Press.
——— . 1995. *Schneider on Schneider: the Conversion of the Jews and Other Anthropological Stories*. Edited by R. Handler. Durham and London: Duke University Press.
——— . 1996 [1969]. 'Kinship, Nationality and Religion in American Culture: Toward a Definition of Kinship', in W. Sollors (ed.), *Theories of Ethnicity: A Classical Reader*. New York: New York University Press, pp. 282–93.
Schweitzer, P. (ed.). 2000. *Dividends of Kinship: Meanings and Uses of Social Relatedness*. New York and London: Routledge.
Segalen, M. 1991. *Fifteen Generations of Bretons: Kinship and Society in Lower Brittany 1720–1980*, trans. J.A. Underwood. Cambridge: Cambridge University Press.
Selbonne, F. 1931. *Contribution à l'étude de la télégonie*. Paris: Lavergne.
Shapin, S. 1996. *The Scientific Revolution*. Chicago: University of Chicago Press.
Shaw, A. 1999. '"What Are 'They' Doing to Our Food?": Public Concerns About Food in the UK', *Sociological Research Online* 4 (3).
——— . 2002. '"It Just Goes Against the Grain." Public Understandings of Genetically Modified (GM) Food in the UK', *Public Understanding of Science* 11 (3): 273–91.
Siebert, C. 1995. 'The DNA We've Been Dealt', *New York Times Magazine*, 17 September.
Silver, L.H. 2001. 'Confused Meanings of Life, Genes and Parents', *Studies in the History and Philosophy of Biology and Biomedical Sciences* 32 (4): 647–61.
Simpson, R. 1994. 'Bringing the "Unclear" Family into Focus: Divorce and Remarriage in Contemporary Britain', *Journal of the Royal Anthropological Institute* (NS) 29: 831–51.
——— . 1998. *Changing Families: an Ethnographic Approach to Divorce and Separation*. Oxford and New York: Berg.
——— . 2004. 'Impossible Gifts: Bodies, Buddhism and Bioethics in Contemporary Sri Lanka', *Journal of the Royal Anthropological Institute* (NS) 10: 839–59.
Siskind, J. 1973. *To Hunt in the Morning*. New York: Oxford University Press.
Sissa, G. 1989. '*Arche Kinousa* ou le paternel comme principe', in *Le Père. Métaphore paternelle et fonctions du père: l'interdit, la filiation, la transmission*. Paris: Denoël, pp. 147–60.
Skultans, V.1998. *The Testimony of Lives. Narrative and Memory in Post-Soviet Latvia*. London and New York: Routledge.
Sökefeld, M. 1999. 'Debating Self, Identity, and Culture in Anthropology', *Current Anthropology* 40 (4): 417–47.
Solberg, B. 2003. 'Etikken i å si nei til sorteringssamfunnet', *Genialt* 2: 20–24.
Sørensen, Ø. and B. Stråth. 1997. 'Introduction', in Ø. Sørensen and B. Stråth (eds), *The Cultural Construction of Norden*. Oslo: Scandinavian University Press, pp. 1–24.
Stacey, J. 1991. *Brave New Families: Stories of Domestic Upheaval in Late Twentieth Century America*. New York: Basic Books.

Sterett, S.M. 2002. 'Introductory Essay', *Law and Society Review* 36 (2): 209–26.
Stevenson, M. 1920. *The Rites of the Twice Born*. London: Oxford University Press.
Stewart, S. 1993. *On Longing: Narratives of the Miniature, the Gigantic, the Souvenir, the Collection*. Durham: Duke University Press.
Stolcke, V. 1986. 'New Reproductive Technologies – Same Old Fatherhood', *Critique of Anthropology* 6: 5–31.
Stone, L. 2000. *Kinship and Gender: an Introduction*, 2nd edn. Boulder: Westview Press.
Strathern, M. 1981. *Kinship at Core: an Anthropology of Elmdon, a Village in North-west Essex in the Nineteen Sixties*. Cambridge: Cambridge University Press.
_____. 1988. *The Gender of the Gift*. Berkeley: University of California Press.
_____. 1992a. *After Nature: English Kinship in the Late Twentieth Century*. Cambridge: Cambridge University Press.
_____. 1992b. *Reproducing the Future: Anthropology, Kinship and the New Reproductive Technologies*. Manchester: Manchester University Press.
_____. 1995. 'Displacing Knowledge: Technology and the Consequences for Kinship', in D. Ginsburg and R. Rapp (eds), *Conceiving the New World Order: the Global Politics of Reproduction*. Berkeley, Los Angeles and London: University of California Press, pp. 346–63.
_____. 1997a. 'Marilyn Strathern on Kinship (Interview with Marilyn Strathern)', *EASA Newsletter* 19: 6–9.
_____. 1997b. 'The Work of Culture: an Anthropological Perspective', in A. Clarke and E. Parsons (eds), *Culture, Kinship and Genes. Towards Cross-Cultural Genetics*. London: Macmillan, pp. 40–53.
_____. 1999. *Property, Substance and Effect*. London: Athlone Press.
_____. 2004. *Commons and Borderland. Working Papers on Interdisciplinarity, Accountability and the Flow of Knowledge*. Wantage: Sean Kingston Publishing.
_____. 2005. *Kinship, Law and the Unexpected. Relatives Are Always a Surprise*. Cambridge: Cambridge University Press.
Teichman, J. 1982. *Illegitimacy: a Philosophical Examination*. Oxford: Blackwell.
Telfer, J.R. 1999. 'Relationship with No Body? "Adoption" Photographs, Intuition and Emotion', *Social Analysis* 43: 144–58.
The President's Council on Bioethics. *Human Cloning and Human Dignity: an Ethical Enquiry*. Washington, D.C., July 2002.
Thiessen, I. 1999. 'The Essence of Being: Procreation and Sexuality in Mid-century Macedonia', in P. Loizos and P. Heady (eds), *Conceiving Persons: Ethnographies of Procreation, Fertility and Growth*. London and New Brunswick, NJ: Athlone Press, pp. 177–200.
Thompson, C. 2001. 'Strategic Naturalizing: Kinship in an Infertility Clinic', in S. Franklin and S. McKinnon (eds), *Relative Values. Reconsidering Kinship Studies*. Durham: Duke University Press, pp. 175–202.
Thompson, E.P. 1993. 'The Moral Economy of the English Crowd in the Eighteenth Century', in *Customs in Common: Studies in Traditional Popular Culture*. New York: New Press, pp. 185–258.
Thorne, B. and M. Yalom. 1992. *Rethinking the Family: Some Feminist Questions*. Boston: Northeastern University Press.
Trägårdh, L. 1997. 'Statist Individualism: On the Culturality of the Nordic Welfare State', in Ø. Sørensen and B. Stråth (eds), *The Cultural Construction of Norden*. Oslo: Scandinavian University Press, pp. 253–85.
Turner, A. 2000. 'Embodied Ethnography. Doing Culture', *Social Anthropology* 8 (1): 51–60.

Tyler, K. 2005. 'The Genealogical Imagination: the Inheritance of Interracial Identities', *The Sociological Review* 53 (3): 475–94.
——— . 2007. 'Race, Genetics and Inheritance: Reflections upon the Birth of "Black" Twins to a "White" IVF Mother', in P. Wade (ed.) *Race, Ethnicity and Nation: Perspectives from Kinship and Genetics*. New York and Oxford: Berghahn Books, pp. 33–51.
Verdery, K. 1999. 'Fuzzy Property: Rights, Power and Identity in Transylvania's Decollectivization', in M. Burawoy and K. Verdery (eds), *Uncertain Transition: Ethnographies of Change in the Postsocialist World*. Lanham, Boulder, New York and Oxford: Rowman and Littlefield, pp. 53–81.
Vernier, B. 1999. *Le Visage et le nom. Contribution à l'étude des systèmes de parenté*. Paris: Presses Universitaires de France.
Wade, P. 2002. *Race, Nature and Culture: An Anthropological Approach*. London: Pluto Press.
——— . (ed.) 2007. *Race, Ethnicity and Nation in Europe: Perspectives from Kinship and Genetics*. New York and Oxford: Berghahn Books.
Wagner, R. 1977. 'Analogic Kinship: a Daribi Example', *American Ethnologist* 4 (4): 623–42.
Wanner, C. 1998. *Burden of Dreams. History and Identity in Post-Soviet Ukraine*. Pennsylvania: State University Press.
Warnock, M. 1985. *A Question of Life. The Warnock Report on Fertilisation and Embryology*. Oxford: Blackwell.
Wert, G., R.T. Meulen, R. Mordacci and M. Tallachini. 2003. *Ethics and Genetics*. Oxford: Berghahn Books.
Westermarck, E. 1901. *The History of Human Marriage*. New York: Macmillan.
Weston, K. 1991. *Family We Choose. Lesbians, Gays, Kinship*. New York: Columbia University Press.
Williams, P. 1981. 'La société', in J.P. Liégeois (ed.), *Les Populations tsiganes en France*. Paris: Centre de recherches tsiganes, Université de Paris V, pp. 27–44.
Wolfram, S. 1987. *In-Laws and Outlaws. Kinship and Marriage in England*. London and Sidney: Croom Helm.
Woolfson, A. 2004. *An Intelligent Person's Guide to Genetics*. London: Duckworth Overlook.
World Value Survey on Hungary. Retrieved 7 November 2005 from http://www.worldvaluessurvey.org/services/index.html.
Wynne, B. 2001. 'Creating Public Alienation: Expert Cultures of Risk and Ethics on GMOs', *Science as Culture* 10 (4): 445–81.
Xanthakou, M. 2000. 'Une histoire pas comme il faut', in J.L. Jamard, E. Terray and M. Xanthakou (eds), *En Substances: Textes pour Françoise Héritier*. Paris: Fayard, pp. 311–28.
Yanagisako, S.J. and J.F. Collier. 1987. 'Toward a Unified Analysis of Gender and Kinship', in J.F. Collier and S.J. Yanagisako (eds), *Gender and Kinship: Essays toward a Unified Analysis*. Stanford: Stanford University Press, pp. 14–50.
Yearbook of Welfare Statistics, 2004. Budapest: Hungarian Central Statistical Office.
Young, M. 1971. *Fighting with Food: Leadership, Values and Social Control in a Massim Society*. Cambridge: Cambridge University Press.
Zonabend, F. 2000. 'Le "dit" et le "lu" de l'inceste', in J.L. Jamard, E. Terray and M. Xanthakou (eds), *En Substances: Textes pour Françoise Héritier*. Paris: Fayard, pp. 289–98.

AUTHOR INDEX

Alber, E., 40
Albie, E., 176
Allison, A., 50–1
Anagnost, A., 75, 76
Aristotle, 106, 125
Astuti, R., 30, 31, 43

Bachelard, G., 97, 99
Barth, F., 32
Bayne, T., 141
Berdahl, D., 31
Bestard, J., 1, 9, 14, 20, 24, 27, 30, 41, 101, 124, 187–8, 191, 193, 194
Boas, F., 49
Bock, J.D., 135
Boholm, Å., 30, 32, 39
Boltanski, L., 92
Bomann-Larsen, T., 144–5
Borneman, J., 14, 148
Bourdieu, P., 32, 171
Broberg, G., 152

Cadoret, A., 2, 6–7, 14, 13, 44n, 80, 109, 148, 151, 159, 183, 184, 188
Calero, L., 120
Campbell, B., 15, 60, 184, 194
Caplan, P., 48, 50
Carson, R., 168
Carsten, J., 2, 5, 9, 11, 15, 30, 43, 51, 56, 97, 117, 181, 187
Cartwright, L., 75
Čepaitienė, A., 10, 31, 39, 182, 188, 190
Changeux, J.P., 193
Clifford, J., 30
Coetzee, J.M., 176

Coghlan, A., 169
Cohen, A., 1, 30
Collier, J.F., 81, 90
Conte, E., 123
Coontz, S., 135
Counihan, C., 49, 56
Cousin, C., 123
Cussins, C., 35

Damien, P., 83
Darr, A., 182
Darwin, C., 119, 166, 173, 176
Dauksas, D., 31, 32
Davison, C., 182
Degnen, C., 7, 12, 57, 110, 181
Delaney, C., 41, 104, 105, 126
Demény, E., 13–4, 110, 150, 157, 189
Descola, P., 163, 165–6, 171, 176, 177
Devereux, C., 173
de Varigny, H., 123
Dooley, D., 187
Dorfles, G., 99
Douaire-Marsaudon, F., 117
Douglas, M., 50, 107
Durant, J., 183
Durkheim, E., 181
Du Bois, C., 48–9

Edwards, J., 9, 14, 19, 29, 30, 31, 32, 35, 39–40, 43, 44n, 45–6, 55–6, 61, 101, 112, 121, 124, 125, 169–70, 182, 187, 195
Elster, J., 99
Essner, C., 123
Evans, J.H., 20

Evans-Pritchard, E.E., 163

Faubion, J., 2
Featherstone, K., 11–2
Feeley-Harnik, G., 163, 166, 173–4
Feinberg, R., 8
Fineman, M.A., 134
Finkler, K., 11, 26, 71, 114
Firbank, L., 171–2
Fortier, C., 104
Foucault, M., 14, 83–4, 130–2, 147, 183, 183–4
Fourmont, M., 100
Franklin, S., 2, 3, 11, 12, 30, 61, 97, 98, 112, 113, 164, 172, 175
Freud, S., 65, 78
Fukuyama, F., 177

García Marín, J.M., 114
Gay y Blasco, P., 107, 108
Geertz, C., 30
Gibbons, D., 169
Gmeiner, H., 129–30
Godelier, M., 194
Goodenough, W.H., 192
Goody, J., 164
Green, S., 47
Grove-White, R., 57
Gudeman, S., 77
Gullestad, M., 1

Haimes, E., 155
Haraway, D., 10, 47–8, 60, 61, 165, 170
Hardardóttir, K.E., 27
Harris, C.C., 4, 8
Hastrup, K., 31, 32
Hayden, C., 2
Heller, C., 57, 58
Helmreich, S., 164, 165
Héritier, F., 15, 37, 83, 97, 110, 117, 123, 126
Hermida, X., 99
Hertz, R., 135
Hervik, P., 31, 32
Hill, J.H., 32
Hirsch, E., 33, 35, 40
Hocart, A., 115
Hoffman-Reim, C., 76
Holy, L., 2, 4, 15, 29, 39

Howell, S., 2, 7, 8, 9, 10, 12, 30, 41, 65, 67, 74, 75, 115, 136, 145, 146, 147, 148, 151, 157, 164, 187, 188

Ingold, T., 173
Ingvaldsen, S., 150, 151, 152, 153

Jacob, F., 20
Jasanoff, S., 10
Jeudi-Ballini, M., 117
Jones, S., 135, 165

Kahn, S.M., 120, 148
Kapitány, B., 132
Knorr-Cetina, K., 10
Kolers, A., 141
Konrad, M., 3, 22, 126, 187, 189
Krusiewicz, E.S., 71, 76
Kuper, A., 118, 119
Kusturica, 174

Labby, D., 117
Lagunas Arias, D., 102, 108
Latour, B., 10, 19–20, 174
Leach, E., 80, 116–7
Leaf, M.J., 193
Legrand, C., 98, 115
Leira, A., 153
Leitch, A., 50
Lévai, 132
Lévi-Strauss, C., 37, 49, 81, 97–8, 168, 173, 179, 184
Levidow, L., 57
Lewin, E., 2
Lezaun, J., 58
Le Roy Ladurie, E., 117–8
Lindee, M.S. 187, 192
Lippman, A., 11
Løvset, J., 153

Malinowski, B., 66
Mannheim, B., 32
Manrique, N., 10, 40, 109, 181, 184
Marre, D., 9, 41, 67, 74, 187, 188, 190
Martin, E., 4, 40, 126
Martínez, A., 68
McKinley, R., 194

McKinnon, S., 2, 11, 164
Melhuus, M., 3, 7, 8, 10, 12, 30, 41, 65, 115, 145, 146, 147, 148, 149, 155–6, 158, 187
Mintz, S., 48–9
Miró, A., 67–9
Modell, J., 2, 64–5, 67, 71–2
Molnár, E., 132
Moore, H., 131
Morgan, L.H., 163, 166
Morley, E., 168, 169
Moscovici, S., 130
Murcott, A., 57, 58
Myerson, G., 48

Nash, C., 13
Needham, R., 4, 115, 116
Nelkin, D., 187, 192
Neményi, M., 132
Nowotny, H., 183

Orobitg, G., 30, 40, 188–90
Ortiz, A.M., 100
Ottenheimer, M., 8

Pálsson, G., 27
Parkin, R., 2, 6, 8, 30
Pasqualino, C., 105
Paukštytė, R., 34
Peirce, C.S., 76
Peletz, M.G., 29
Pereiro, X.M., 99
Pina-Cabral, J., 77
Plato, 97
Pliny, 77
Pocius, G.L., 32
Pollan, M., 176
Pollock, C., 167
Pongrácz, T., 132
Porqueres i Gené, E., 3, 5, 13, 15, 37, 101, 118, 180

Rabinow, P., 46–7, 61, 180
Radcliffe-Brown, A.R., 168, 174
Ragoné, H., 3, 29, 35, 188
Rapp, R., 180, 188
Rappaport, R.A., 163
Rausing, S., 31
Read, D.W., 194
Rheinberger, H.J., 20

Richards, M., 182
Ricoeur, P., 32, 131
Roll-Hansen, N., 152
Rønne-Pettersen, E., 153
Roscoe, P.B., 100
Rose, S., 147
Rylott, P., 168, 169

Sahlins, M., 116
Salazar, C., 2, 13, 30, 43, 93, 140, 185, 189, 194
Sandemose, A., 153
Scheffler, H.W., 18n27
Schneider, D., 1–2, 6, 7, 8, 11, 12, 13, 28, 30, 32, 37, 39, 43, 52, 80, 113, 115–7, 140, 164, 191,
Schweitzer, P., 131–2
Segalen, M., 30
Shapin, S., 183
Shaw, A., 57, 58
Silver, L.H., 181
Silverman, S., 11
Simpson, R., 2, 34, 35
Siskind, J., 49
Sissa, G., 125
Skultans, V., 30–1
Sökefeld, M., 31
Sørensen, O., 148
Souto, M., 121
Stacey, J., 2
Sterett, S.M., 147
Stevenson, M., 114
Stewart, S., 76
Stone, L., 2, 6, 8, 30
Stråth, B., 148
Strathern, M., 1, 3–4, 6, 9, 13, 19, 22, 26, 28, 29, 30, 31, 32, 35, 39, 40, 43, 82, 83, 97, 112, 113–4, 163, 164, 180, 191
Streicher, J., 123

Taussig, K.S., 11
Teichman, J., 149, 150
Telfer, J.R., 66–7, 75, 76
Thiessen, I., 34
Thompson, C., 3, 124, 165
Thorne, B., 131
Trägårdh, L., 148
Turner, A., 32

Verdery, K., 31
Vernier, B., 65

Wade, P., 1, 3
Wanner, C., 31
Wert, G., 179
Westermarck, E., 100
Weston, K., 2

Wilgaux, J., 3, 5, 13, 15, 37, 101, 180, 181
Wolfram, S., 118
Wood, J.T., 71, 76
Woolfson, A., 176, 177

Yalom, M., 131
Yanagisako, S.J., 81, 90
Young, M., 49

SUBJECT INDEX

abortion, 114, 190
actor network theory (ANT), 14
Adam and Eve, 38
Adoption, 12
   of animals, 174
   anonymity and, 153–4, 157–8, 187
   in Catalonia, 64–78
   in China, 72–4
   kinship and, 149, 159
   matching, 72–4
   in Norway, 74, 146, 147–53, 156–8
   transnational, 8, 12, 14, 41, 77, 67–8, 113–5, 164, 149, 155, 157, 159, 188
   versus gamete donation, 147, 154
AID (artificial insemination by donor) *see* artificial insemination
anonymity *see under* adoption; artificial insemination
ANT *see* actor network theory (ANT)
anthropology, 11, 80
   formal analysis, 193
   intellectualist, 182–3
   see also kinship; knowledge; structuralism
anti-semitism, 123
ART (assisted reproductive technologies) *see* assisted reproductive technologies
artificial insemination, 40, 41, 80, 85–6, 87, 90–3, 114, 120–1, 124, 144–6, 153–5, 158, 188
   anonymity and, 21–3, 154–5, 157–8, 187
assisted reproductive technologies (ART), 8, 20, 21–34, 40, 42–3, 66, 81, 134–5, 155
   family and, 162
   illegitimacy and, 149
   see also artificial insemination; egg (ova), donation of; new reproductive technologies
Australia, 121–2
Austria, 120

Bali, 116
belonging *see* adoption; artificial insemination; egg donation; gamete donation
best interest of the child *see* child, best interest of
Bible, 38
biodiversity, 168–74, 180
bioethics, 179
biogenetic inheritance, 69–71, 77–8
biologisation, 11, 27, 145, 188
biology, 3–4, 6, 8, 12–3
biosociality, 46–7, 60–1, 180
biotechnology, 11–2, 45, 46, 50, 166, 169, 170, 177
birds, 166–9, 173–5
blood, 9–10, 13, 23, 27, 98–9, 117, 125–6, 181
   'bad', 106–7
   genes and, 5, 6
   among Gypsies, 101–110
   in Lithuania, 36–7
'boundary objects', 169–70
breast-feeding, 51–2

cannibalism, 117
Castberg Children's Acts, 150

Catalonia, 21–8, 64–78
Catholic Church, 118–9, 122–4
Chernobyl, 34
child, 34–6, 38–9, 41–2
  best interest of, 150, 152, 159
  rights of, 149, 157–8
China, 72–4
Christianity *see* Catholic Church
concubinage, 118
consanguinity, 118–23, 180–1
  see also incest
consubstantiality, 117, 126, 180–1

divorce, 36
DNA, 180, 187
dogs, 165
donation eggs *see* egg (ova), donation of
donor insemination *see* artificial insemination

egg (ova)
  donation of, 21–8, 115, 124–5, 149, 155–6, 188–9, 191
  incest and, 121
  oocyte, 21, 23, 24
embryo
  Franklin on, 113–4
  frozen, 12, 121
  Human Fertilisation and Embryology Act (Britain, 1990), 113, 176
  rights of, 114
  visualisation of, 70, 113
  see also fetus
Enlightenment, 83, 164, 165, 183
essentialism, 26
ethnography, 28
eugenics, 119, 151–2
Euro-American, 6–8, 28

'facts of life', 181
family
  AID and, 153
  homoparental, 80, 85–96, 113
  in Hungary, 132–6
  nuclear, 134
father, 134–5
feminism, 5

fetus
  among Gypsies, 104
  rights of, 114
  see also embryo
filiation, 184
folk model, 6, 7, 8
food, 7, 48–9, 181
  children and, 52–6
  Genetically Modified Food (GMF), 7, 12, 45–50, 54–62
  in Japan, 51
  in Malaysia, 51–2
  organic, 54–5
foster care, 13–4
foster mothers *see* motherhood, foster

gametes, 3, 7
  donation of, 20–8, 40, 42, 77, 124
  donation versus adoption, 147, 154
  see also artificial insemination; egg
genes, 27, 98–9, 110, 117, 126, 180
  blood and, 5, 6, 125–6
  genetic modification, 163–4
  identity and, 83–4, 121
  kinship and, 191–5
  uniqueness of, 180
Genetically Modified Food (GMF), 7, 12, 45–50, 54–62
Genetically Modified Organisms (GMO), 15, 166–77, 184
geneticisation, 11–2, 14, 26–8
Genetics, 13
  public understanding of (PUG), 1, 20, 28, 142, 160, 183
  as relational, 179–80
  as truth knowledge, 185–7, 190–1
genome *see* human genome
GMF *see* Genetically Modified Food
GMO *see* Genetically Modified Organisms

heredity *see* biogenetic inheritance
Human Fertilisation and Embryology Act (Britain, 1990), 113
human genome, 20, 47, 98
Hungary, 119–22, 128–43, 150
husband, 35–7, 122

Index

identity, 65, 83–4, 121, 131
  genes and, 83–4, 121
  Moore on, 131
illegitimacy, 149, 150, 152, 185
in vitro fertilisation (IVF), 155, 158, 177, 188
incest, 5, 115–26
  in Australia, 121–2
  in Austria, 120
  brother/sister, 99–100, 112
  in Hungary, 119–22
  new genetics and, 112–27
  Schneider on, 115–6
  'of second type' (Héritier), 123
  taboo as universal, 126
  among Yapese, 116–7
infertility, 34–5, 38, 153–4
international adoption *see* adoption, transnational
Ireland, 191
IVF *see in vitro* fertilisation

Japan, 51
Jews, 31–2

'kinning', 158, 164, 170
kinship
  anthropology and, 11, 80
  as analytical tool, 19
  biology and, 3–4, 8, 12
  children and, 34–6, 38–9, 42
  as defunct (Franklin), 112–3
  fictive, 3
  genes and, 13, 180–1, 191–5
  in Lithuania, 33–4
  'materiality of', 8
  NRT and, 162–3
  'odour' of, 83
  plural, 15
  post-human, 163–4, 166, 175
  as relational, 162–3
  resemblance and, 64–78
  social relations and, 181
  as symbolic knowledge, 185–7, 190–1
  as 'thinking', 46
  Western/European, 8
knowledge, 184
  social/asocial, 184–5

syntagmatic/paradigmatic, 184
truth/symbol, 185–7, 190–1

Lithuania, 29–44
local thinking/imaginings, 30–1

Malaysia, 51–2
matching *see under* adoption
meaning/truth, 184
medicalisation, 114
menstruation (menses), 103–6, 108–10
metaphor/metonymy, 173, 190, 194
  see also knowledge, syntagmatic/paradigmatic
mothers
  birth, 185–7
  foster, 14, 128–42, 185, 189
  surrogate, 3, 9–10, 18n27, 42
  symbolic, 190

naming, 6–7
  adoption and, 151
  foster mothers and, 131
  lesbian parents and, 88–9
  law (in Norway) on, 151
nature, 81, 153, 182, 183
Nazism, 153
Neothomism, 119
networks, 14, 19
new genetics, 112
new reproductive technologies (NRT), 1, 3, 8, 11–2, 14, 76, 124, 146–9, 152–6, 159
  see also assisted reproductive technologies (ART)
Norway 9, 10, 41
  adoption laws, 150–5
  royalty, 144–5
NRT *see* new reproductive technologies (NRT)

'odel', 152
Olav, King, 144–6, 148
oocyte, 21, 23, 24
organic food *see* food, organic
ova *see* egg (ova)

parents, 151
  lesbian, 5, 15, 85–96

pater est, 148, 153
payo, 103, 107–8
pets, 165–6
pigeons, 173, 174
post-humanism, 163–4, 166, 175, 177
postmodernism, 5, 164
procreation, 109–10
psychoanalysis *see* Freud
public understanding of genetics (PUG) *see* genetics, public understanding of (PUG)
PUG *see* genetics, public understanding of (PUG)

racial hygiene, 153
relationality, 126, 162–3, 179–80, 195

Samoa, 116
science, 10–11, 182–3, 185
semen, 14, 15, 125
  donation of *see* artificial insemination
  Gypsies on, 103–6, 109–10, 181
sexual intercourse, 102–3, 180–1
  SOS Children's Villages, 128–30, 133–42, 189

sperm *see* semen
structuralism, 164
  see also Lévi-Strauss in name index
subject/object, 47–8
surrogacy, 3, 9–10, 18n27, 124–5
symbols *see* knowledge; totemism
syntagmatic/paradigmatic, 184, 194

technoscience, 47–8, 61–2
telegony, 123–4
tomato, 177
  transgenic, 47
totemism, 168, 173
transnational adoption *see* adoption, transnational
truth
  Foucault on, 83–4, 183–4
  truth/meaning, 184
  see also knowledge

Una Caro, 122

vivisection, 174

Warnock Report (1985), 120
wife, 35–7, 122
World Trade Organisation (WTO), 166